Healing the Eating Habit
Sofia Bothwell
Copyright Sofia Bothwell 2023
ISBN 978-1-4477-7315-3

Disclaimer: The author of this book does not dispense medical, psychological or psychiatric advice nor prescribes the use of any technique as a form of treatment for medical problems without the advice of a physician. Your health and the advice you take is, as always, to be done through your own discernment and is your complete responsibility.

Sofia Bothwell

# INTRODUCTION

It is more than a decade since I healed my own eating disorder. I am eternally grateful that I am no longer a compulsive eater. In this book, I share with you the ideas, knowledge and insights that enable me to be healed today.
I am sitting in the small, bright sitting room of the West Hampstead flat I call home, eagerly starting to write this manuscript. It is a hot, glorious London summer. The summer is alive, like a force all of its own, oblivious to the hum drum lives and dramas of the cosmopolitan inhabitants of this city. I am lucky to be one of them, an Irish immigrant just starting her first self-help support groups for compulsive eating women in a local holistic centre. I breathe, and am aware of the warmth of the room, the distant sounds of a radio, the lush green of nature majestically swaying and rustling in unseen breezes.
I am yet again reminded, that six months ago I watched snow lying on this same landscape. What a transformation! A huge transformation comprised of a million tiny steps of gradual progression. Who could define those tiny changes which, all added together, comprise the evolution from winter bleakness to summer abundance?
I often think of nature as the perfect metaphor for what we all do as we involve ourselves in the personal growth and self-

healing process. Affirmations repeated, are the drops of rain, nurturing a seed to growth. A goal visualised, is the dream of summer, dreamt in winter. A written goal and a plan for achieving it is the snow-laden tree, which produces small green buds, small green leaves, and then a mass of fully mature leaves which rustle and sway in the glory of a goal accomplished.

Blossoms, the prerequisite to fruit, are the daily times of meditation where peace and beauty are found and later lead to the fruit of healthy relationships and a satisfying life. The daily practice of forgiveness and release is the fertile soil in which the seeds of abundance flourish and grow.

The first light green haze of newly opened buds, like mists enveloping the woods and forests, are the hushed whispers from our higher selves, calling us to heal and guiding us, on our way.

## How 'Healing the Eating Habit' got its name

When I started working in the field of personal development and healing, catchy meaningful titles accompanied most workshops available. A good idea. A title that concisely sums up your work leaves everyone instantly clear about the workshop content.

I had advertised my work under various headings such as: 'Weight Loss Is Easy!' And, 'Is Weight and Food a Constant Concern?' All perfectly good titles but I felt they lacked a certain Oomph. It seemed as if the New Age had just hit London. Many famous American authors were doing lectures and workshops here, enlightening all before them! I was enthused, and felt

privileged to be part of a growing awareness of light and healing. A multilevel, conscious evolving for the planet.
So, with such dynamic forces at play I felt it was my duty to live up to the highest expectations of me. A few people had already asked me – 'What's your workshop called?' And my reply was – 'I don't have a name for it yet, but if you think of something appropriate, I'd appreciate you letting me know!' Time passed and still 'no name' workshops were doing well. I had already started putting this hand written manuscript on my computer, and was tentatively realising that my dream of writing a book was in fact unfolding before my eyes. Then, it came to me – the title for my book! – Healing the Eating Habit! The title was held in my mind. Clear and definite. I felt so good about discovering an appropriate name for my book that I typed on my computer, in big, bold italic letters – Healing the Eating Habit!

At that time I was happily expecting my first baby, and I began to take on one to one sessions as well as my weekly support groups / workshops. I thought about using my new found book title as an overall title for the process I was teaching. I thought about the word 'habit.' A habit is a learned response, a settled tendency or practice, certainly something that can be altered, improved on or even changed completely. That seemed to describe exactly what I was doing in my work. Yes, I was certainly dealing with habits and the business of changing them. Even more appropriately, the word habit is sometimes attached to the idea of addiction. Now more than ever I wanted to convey the idea, that a person who regularly eats even though they are physically full – is a food addict.

What I had experienced when I overcame my own eating disorder some ten years previously in 1983, was definitely the conquering of my addiction to food and it was more. More than a conquering, more than changing. It was a healing.

Through reading Susie Orbach's book Fat Is A Feminist Issue and following through on her ideas and guidelines, I had been able to completely transform my eating habits from those of a compulsive eater, to those that are completely in harmony with my body's own hunger and fullness sensations. What I had experienced with great relief was a true and complete healing. I said to myself – Yes, this healing is what I want other women to know and experience for themselves. The more I thought about it, the more I felt how perfect it was to call my book and my work in individual sessions and workshops – Healing the Eating Habit.

**Ask yourself** and several of your friends: 'Are you completely accepting of and satisfied with your size and shape?' Prepare yourself for a few negative responses! The point I would like to emphasise here is this: Most people are not at all accepting of, nor satisfied with, what they have the most intimate of connections with – their own bodies. Changing this lack of self-acceptance is one of the first important steps in healing your eating habit.

In this book we shall look at the role of self-acceptance, along with how, and why to develop it. I will show you how to learn the difference between emotional and physical hunger. We shall look at emotional issues and how to resolve them. All this and more is explored in the following pages, in an effort to understand and conquer this modern day scourge, which is addiction to food, and obsession with size, shape and appearance. Where the obsessive behaviour comes from, how it manifests and how to heal it permanently, will all be covered, so you can gain greater knowledge of what makes you the person you are and how to change the bits you want to change.

To be a food addict and to want to overcome the 'food thing' is a position in which many women find themselves today. Reading a self-help book such as this one, joining a support group, or forming one, will all help you kick your overeating habit. This book is very much a step in the right direction. I congratulate you for having the courage to face up to your eating habits and weight problems, and to tackle the underlying emotional root cause of overeating and binge eating. I am delighted to share with you the concepts and tools which enabled me to recover and stay recovered from my own eating disorder and emerge, with relief, into a world where food holds no fear; and a natural, truly nurturing and pleasurable relationship to food replaces an addicted one.

Breaking the negative cycle of compulsive eating is possible. Sometimes, it needs persistence. Always, it requires a true desire to get better. Using the tools that appeal to you, and with the support of good friends, a support group or therapist, you do find your way to a completely healthy and natural relationship to food. This evolves as the natural result of following these three guidelines:

1.  The awareness of when physically hungry and physically full, and acting appropriately on those inner cues.
2.  Raising self-acceptance.
3.  Pinpointing and resolving emotional issues rather than suppressing them.

These are the three major guidelines, which enable us to lose any excess weight and maintain that weight loss permanently. Following these guidelines is our main objective now. The loss of excess weight, naturally and permanently, results for anyone who has these three guidelines operating in their lives. Let's consider each one of these guidelines in detail.

## Guideline 1

<u>The awareness of when physically hungry and physically full, and acting appropriately on those inner cues.</u> This means knowing when you are genuinely physically hungry and eating at that point. Knowing when you are genuinely physically full and being able to stop eating at that point. Knowing what emotional hunger is, what it feels like and knowing what to do when it strikes!

All this may seem like the simplest thing in the world to do, but believe me, it can be the most difficult if you are a compulsive eater. However, with the right knowledge, practical tools and practice, healing your compulsive eating habit can be successfully accomplished.

## So what is emotional hunger?

Emotional hunger is the craving to eat even though you are already physically full. The sensation of emotional hunger is experienced in the mouth rather than the stomach. Often referred to as mouth hunger, there is a distinct difference between this craving or compulsion to eat when full and the healthy desire to eat as a result of genuine physical hunger. The difference between these two 'hunger states' is what you will be familiarising yourself with in the first few weeks and months of healing your eating habit. This can be a very rewarding and interesting time.

## What to do about emotional hunger?

In order to be able to stop eating when physically full it is necessary to know how to handle emotional hunger. Here's how:

Respond to emotional hunger by first of all tuning into your feelings. You can do this by asking yourself one or all of the following questions:

What feeling is this?

What emotion am I experiencing now?

What emotional issue or problem is this about?

What words can best describe how I am feeling right now?

Is this feeling 'held' somewhere in my body?

Can I feel an emotional sensation anywhere in my body?
Secondly, whilst allowing yourself to experience your feelings, ask yourself this all-important question:
Given the fact I feel this way, what would I like to do now?
And then, get busy doing it! Knowing this (i.e. what you would like to do, at that moment in time, when you are physically full but still crave to eat more) is the means by which you break out of those old negative eating patterns. For the answer to this all-important question is, the healthy alternative to stuffing down the feelings. When you get busy doing this healthy alternative, you are meeting your emotional needs appropriately, rather than stuffing them down with food when full. And you are well on the way to healing your eating habit completely. Please remember when asking yourself the question – Given the fact I feel this way, what would I like to do now? – that it is - What would I like to do now? Not - What should I do?

I should be cleaning the kitchen, mowing the lawn or de-fleeing the cat but what I would like to do is probably something completely different and much more likely to meet my emotional needs.

**Example:** You have just finished eating a hot meal which you really enjoyed. You allowed yourself to eat exactly what you wanted and stopped when you were full. You are now sitting in front of the TV. You have just finished a nice cup of coffee and three of your favourite chocolate biscuits. You want to eat more biscuits. You feel the urge to go into the kitchen and find yourself some more of those biscuits to eat. You ask yourself:

Am I physically hungry? The answer is - No. You check in with your stomach, noticing how it feels. It feels full. You notice the craving to continue eating. Now, this is the time to ask yourself: What feeling is this? What emotional issue is this? You notice that you are feeling dissatisfied with your living arrangements and especially your flat mate with whom you have had several arguments. Now that you have realised how you are feeling emotionally (dissatisfied) and what the issue is (whether to get a new place to live or stick it out here) you ask yourself: Given the fact I feel this way, what would I like to do now? You look around and realise that you have grown somewhat tired of your flat. You notice that you have a strong desire to move out and even though fear has always stopped you in the past, you resolve to look for a new flat.

Thus the answers to – What feeling is this? And – Given the fact I feel this way, what would I like to do now? – are very valuable for they provide you with an appropriate alternative to eating when physically full and help you resolve an important emotional issue. It is this alternative way of dealing with your feelings, which allows you to experience, resolve and integrate your feelings easily, and cease eating compulsively in order to suppress your feelings and emotional issues.

The practice of asking – What feeling is this? And – Given the fact I feel this way, what would I like to do now? And following up on the healthy answer, further enables you to resolve your emotional issues, and thus helps you to stop eating when physically full.

Often I am asked: 'But what if, when I ask myself – 'What would I like to do now?' The answer is – Have a large gin and tonic, or a cigarette, or pick a fight with my husband, or eat ten chocolate biscuits even though I am definitely full?

Well, as you are probably aware, none of these activities are the healthy, ideal alternatives for which you are looking. You know that all these activities, if carried out, would only be abusive to either yourself or your husband, and are just another form of stuffing your feelings down into suppression rather than dealing with them constructively. This is swapping addictions as opposed to resolving the root cause of that addiction, the unresolved emotional issues. So when this temptation to swap addictions arises you can come back to the old reliable question: Given the fact I feel this way what would I like to do now? And follow up on the healthy answer you receive. Thus ensuring that you do not swap your addictions but completely breakthrough your tendencies towards addiction to a healthier way of life.

As you continue on your own personal road to recovery, you will become more and more aware of when you are doing something in order to distance yourself from your feelings. This awareness increases until you are in the constant process of feeling your feelings and acting appropriately on their guidance. The suppression of feelings becomes nothing more than an inadequate means of coping. This can take time to evolve so do not worry if you are not sure right away what is addicted behaviour and what is healthy behaviour. The intention and willingness to be more aware of and open to your own feelings is enough to make great progress in this area. In truth, you are becoming more intuitive.

## Eat when physically hungry

With physical hunger some women tell me: 'But I am never hungry.' They literally, never allow themselves to feel physical hunger. They are always physically full. This is what I recommend to help. One day when you wake up, go without food for three or four hours. After that time you will be able to identify some real, physical hunger sensations, ranging from slightly hungry to very hungry. You can respond to these hunger sensations appropriately by asking yourself: 'What would I like to eat now?' And eating whatever you want, as many different types of food that you want until you are physically full.

Many of you find it difficult to eat outside of mealtimes, or think that you should only eat certain foods at certain times. The breakfast, lunch and dinner regime! In truth, when it comes to healthy eating, once you are physically hungry, it does not matter what time of day it is. Do allow yourself ultimate freedom in terms of what you eat and when you eat, for maximum benefit. Your mealtimes might be a bit array but you will no longer be a food addict. A sensible idea wouldn't you say?

So, let's not delay. If you are really hungry at 12 noon, know that it is ridiculous to wait until regimented mealtime at 2pm before allowing yourself to eat. There is no point in causing yourself the needless discomfort of an empty stomach getting more and more empty, when you could be busily enjoying a tuna sandwich and cappuccino at the local deli.

Be kind and considerate to your stomach, your whole body and self; when you are physically hungry, eat at that moment in time, without delay, and make sure it is what you really fancy eating, and stop when physically full.

## Stop eating when physically full

Sometimes it is difficult to stop eating when physically full. Many women find it almost impossible at first and that's okay, we have a tool to help with this too! Try leaving behind about a spoonful of each type of food on your plate at every meal. This means, leaving a spoonful or two of soup, desert, potatoes, meat, vegetables etc. Simply leave it sitting on your plate and notice how you feel. This practice not only helps you to stop eating when physically full and firmly establish a true and valuable sense of control around food, it can also help you break out of that well known, harmful habit learned in childhood of finishing everything on your plate no matter what!

Leaving food on your plate often brings up painful memories of dysfunctional messages from the past. Do any of the following ring a bell?

'Finish everything on your plate. It is a waste to throw it away.'

'Do you know how much that cost!?'

Statements like these about money and wastage only serve to make us feel guilty and fearful about money. Possibly concluding – There is not enough.

'The time I spent cooking and now you don't want to eat it!' Again guilt is thrown at us.

'You cannot go out and play / leave the table / watch TV until you have finished everything on your plate.' Your wishes not being considered. Control. Negative experience of authority. Possible conclusions – I'm not important, I don't get what I want, my needs aren't important.

'Eat your greens / meat / cheese because they are good for you.' – Being forced to eat food you genuinely did not like the taste of because it would be 'good' for you. Possible conclusion – Things that are good for me are unpleasant. I cannot trust my inner knowing as to what to eat and what not to eat.

'Look at all the starving in the world.' Filling you with guilt and fear.

'You finish your dinner and then you can have desert!' In other words, you are not allowed to eat sweet things before savoury. You are not allowed to eat what you fancy. The order you eat food seems to have more to do with strict social rules and control, than healthy enjoyment and personal choice. Possible conclusion – I can't trust my body to tell me what to eat and when to eat, if it is causing this much commotion. There are silly rules to follow.

Leaving at least a spoonful of food on your plate is demonstrating the fact that your eating habits are no longer governed by these inappropriate echoes of the past. If you are having a bar of chocolate, then leave a small piece of chocolate in the wrapper when you are throwing it in the bin. By all means have another chocolate bar if you are, still physically hungry and it is chocolate you fancy eating; but do remember to leave behind that one mouthful of each bar. Keep doing this with everything you eat, until you gain the feeling that you are in control of the food, rather than the food being in control of you. The compulsion to polish off everything on your plate, even though you are physically full, does dissolve.

## Overindulgence

Now, there may be a certain amount of overindulgence at this early stage of allowing yourself to eat whatever you want, when physically hungry. You may find, that all you want to eat when physically hungry, are the so called fattening foods. You may discover that you go again and again, when physically hungry, for the cakes, crisps, chips, apple pie and cream cakes that you so strictly denied yourself with every diet. This is just a natural factor, balancing forced denial, with overindulgence. So don't worry, if you eat a lot of chocolate when physically hungry, this is simply because you denied yourself chocolate when you were dieting, so you are making up for it now. Know that once you are stopping when physically full, you will not gain weight. At this moment in time, do reassure yourself of the diet-busting truth – No food has the power to make you gain weight unless it is eaten when you are physically full.

It also seems to me to be a testing time. It's as if one part of you is testing the other part of you. It's as if one part of you is saying

– 'Oh yes, I can eat whatever I want once I am physically hungry.' And another part of you tests it by saying – 'Are you sure about that?! I am physically hungry and I fancy chocolate cake.' That part of you is almost expecting to be denied that chocolate cake, and it needs proof that it really can eat whatever it wants until physically full. It is your job, to assure yourself, that you will never again deny yourself your favourite foods when you are physically hungry. And this assurance, comes with, going through an unhealthy food phase, where you are eating when you are physically hungry and practising stopping when physically full, however what you tend to eat when hungry is carbohydrate, sugar or chocolate. An unhealthy mixture you might say. And yes it is an unhealthy food phase. Soon you find that you do not actually want to live off chocolate, or even eat more than one bar a day at the most. However, only permission and allowance of all food creates the climate in which you can make this discovery. You do find, the result of assuring yourself that you can eat whatever you want when physically hungry, is that you want healthier foods. Yes, you will still eat chips, chocolate and cake but you also eat fruit, vegetables, grilled foods and salads. Your food intake becomes a wide variety of foods, savoury, sweet, bland, spicy, fresh, frozen. A perfect balance of the so called healthy and so called unhealthy foods.

When you have a solid assurance, that you are never going to deny yourself chocolate or any of your favourite foods, you dissolve the automatic – 'Well I am jolly well going to eat it and then some!' – reaction to forced denial. Chocolate simply becomes chocolate. A wonderful food with a wonderful taste. One of the many wonderful foods both sweet and savoury that have wonderful tastes, textures and aromas. All of which are allowed.

## A child's right to choose

The old ideas previously mentioned of eating everything on your plate, and *savoury* before *sweet* etc, did not take into account some very important considerations:

1.   Whether or not you were physically full.
2.   What you fancied eating or doing at that moment in time.

In other words you were robbed of your right to choose in the arena of food. Through this lack of choice you were hindered in becoming self-determined in this area. When you did make a choice and demonstrated it by, for example, getting up and leaving the table when you were half way through your plateful of food but physically full – your decision that you were full and wanted to leave the room was overridden by your parent saying – 'Stay here and finish what is on your plate.' No choice. You were full but you had to eat. Much the same feeling after a binge – you were full but you had to eat! Thus you learned how to override your stomach's fullness signals.

To deny a child the right to determine when she starts and finishes eating is inappropriate and harmful because it does not support the child's built in sense of trust in what her own stomach is telling her. Rather the idea that the body's own natural hunger and fullness mechanism cannot be true, and what mother says is true, even if what mother is in fact saying is as ridiculous a notion as – 'Do not stop eating when your stomach says you are full, but keep on stuffing in more food until I say you have had enough or your plate says you have had enough by being empty.' So, the child treated in such a way does not know who to trust, her own stomach sensations, or what mother says. And so you have the present day situation where a grown woman cannot trust what her own stomach is telling her, and refers to the diet sheets (an outer authority like mother) in order to tell her how much, and what, she 'should' be eating. Meanwhile, her stomach has been trying to tell her, just that, all along. However she ignores those very natural and accurate hunger and fullness sensations, just like mother ignored her exclamations of 'But Mum I am full!' So this grown woman is still eating when her stomach is genuinely physically full, and is continuing to eat until her plate is empty. Thus she gains weight, because 'food when full' is 'fattening food.'

That was the painful lesson of the past – Finish everything on your plate - which well-meaning but misguided mothers taught. And which I encourage you to examine and move away from so you can get to the healthy stage of trusting your own hunger and fullness sensations, for they guide you to eat when physically hungry and stop when physically full. They guide you to your own natural weight.

You now know, how you first learned to override your body's natural, healthy inner cues about when to eat and when to stop eating. If your childhood was filled with inappropriate and confusing messages, just notice these old memories when they arise and allow yourself to feel the feelings associated with them. You can affirm for these old memories and feelings — This is over. It is past. It is finished. I now release past painful memories about food and eating, knowing everyone did their best but I now choose another way. I am free to change my eating habits. I forgive everyone who pushed me to eat even though I was physically full. I now allow myself to eat when I am hungry and stop when I am full.

**Listening to my stomach**
It is also good to pause and put down your knife and fork when you are half way through a meal, this provides you with a valuable opportunity to sit back and relax and simply notice your stomach and what it is telling you. At this point, ask yourself — Is my stomach completely full now, or half full? Is there room for a coffee and something sweet? Or am I positively stuffed but have a compulsion to keep on eating? Have I any cravings towards wine or other alcohol? In which case I can ask myself — What feeling is this? And — Given the fact I feel this way what would I like to do now?

**For example:**
Your stomach is full of food and would like you to stop eating so that it can comfortably digest its contents. Or your stomach would like you to stop eating the savoury main course, and round off that meal with a chocolate and a coffee, as you fancy something sweet and have just enough room for it.

## Heavenly State

You may well ask: 'How on earth am I going to lose weight with my sweet tooth and you telling me to eat as much as I want of exactly what I want, even if it is chocolate?' Well the important point which best describes the logic behind, what many would consider to be the heavenly state of being able to eat exactly what we want, when we want, as long as we are physically hungry, is this – The sole cause of excess weight is eating when physically full. It is not so much what we eat, as the eating when physically full that causes weight gain and hinders weight loss.

Remember the all-important condition, physical hunger for it is our gauge; not the echo of our mother's voice, not the latest diet sheet, nor the empty plate. The ultimate authority now in telling us when to eat is our stomach's hunger and fullness sensations. As long as we are physically hungry we can eat whatever we want without fear of weight gain. To only eat when genuinely physically hungry, means we stop eating when physically full. If you eat when physically hungry and stop when physically full you do not gain excess weight, because you have eliminated that which causes the excess weight – the eating when physically full.

## Eating when physically full is the cause of weight gain

With the awareness and resolving of the emotional issues which have previously sent us to the biscuit tin even though we were full, our ability to stop eating when physically full increases until it becomes this natural automatic reaction – I am physically full, I stop eating.

Along with the reassurance that you are now allowing yourself to eat whatever you want, and as much as you want until physically full, comes the dissipation of the urge to binge. Knowing that you can eat whatever you want, whenever you want as long as you are physically hungry, actively challenges the compulsive urge to eat when full. You are allowing yourself abundance. No more forbidden foods. You are adopting the attitude of – 'I've been eating when full for years now, and I could continue to eat when full for the rest of my life. Now do I want to do that, or do I want to do what it takes to empower me to stop? Eating when full could remain my inadequate means of coping with feelings and issues or I could actively seek, find and put into practice the alternatives to eating when full. Now what am I going to choose? Which course of action?

You are in the process of changing your relationship to food from an addicted one to a nurturing one, and you will probably do some eating when full in the first few weeks and months while undertaking this challenging task. However, you are now approaching your eating habits from a whole new angle, and after a few binges you will be even more aware of how physically uncomfortable eating when full really is. You are becoming more and more willing to feel the feelings, that used to drive you to binge to keep suppressed. Overeating has already proven itself to be an inadequate means of coping, and you are now realising that you have a choice. Eat when full or stop eating when full, feel and resolve your feelings by asking yourself and acting on the healthy answer to the question – Given the fact I feel this way what would I like to do now?

## Responsibility Trust Freedom

You are beginning to develop a trust in your body and your ability to meet your body's needs appropriately, both emotional and physical. You are giving yourself permission to eat your favourite foods without restriction. In giving yourself permission comes responsibility, the responsibility to make the right choice – the choice to stop eating when physically full and wait for physical hunger before you eat again. The responsibility to forgive yourself if you do binge. After all, you are trying to change the habit of many years. You are trusting yourself to make that change positive and complete. This is big emotional work. Congratulate yourself for embarking on such a journey into the unknown realm of your own consciousness.

In doing yourself the great favour of healing your own eating habit, you are giving yourself freedom. Freedom from obsession. But remember, awareness and responsibility are the price tags on freedom.

Freedom from obsession is a sign of abundance and plenty, which are the sure forerunners of good health, whereas it is ideas of lack and restriction (remind you of any diet?) that lie the root concepts of addiction and dis-ease. When you know that you can eat exactly what you fancy as long as you are physically hungry, why should you binge? In order to stuff down an emotional issue, you may say. This is true. Hence, the importance of our next guideline - the resolving of the emotional issues which, through eating when physically full, we had kept firmly under wraps.

When eating when physically full occurs, it is a sign that an emotional issue is still unresolved. Occasional eating when full or binge eating can occur in the first few weeks and sometimes months of practising these guidelines, this is simply because there is still unresolved issues for you and you still use *food when full* as your means of dealing with them. If you have a binge, do not beat yourself up about it. After all, it takes longer than a week to resolve everything. With patience and persistence, one by one, your emotional issues emerge from your subconscious and get resolved. You are less inclined to overeat in order to suppress an emotion when that emotion has been resolved.

We do not have the urge or compulsion to binge once the issues have been resolved. Instead, we are busy dealing with our feelings and emotional issues in new more appropriate, enjoyable and healthy ways.

All that is required in order to know when one is physically hungry and when one is physically full, is a general tuning in to one's stomach. In other words, be aware of the physical sensations which are coming from your own stomach. Even if you are in the middle of a meal, you can pause a few times in order to be more aware of that part of your body which does all the digesting and what signals it is sending you in terms of hunger and fulness sensations. Thus, you become familiar with the subtle and pleasurable sensations of a full, contented stomach. Of course if you ignore those subtle signs of physical fullness and continue eating, you are going to get some not-so-subtle signs of discomfort such as indigestion, bloating, nausea or gas. So, in more ways than one, it pays to tune into and obey those sensations of physical hunger and physical fullness.

**Remember:**
When you are physically hungry, ask yourself – What do I fancy eating?
In the middle of eating ask yourself – Am I physically full yet? And do I want to eat more of the same food, or something different?
Eat exactly what you want when you are physically hungry, and practice leaving at least a spoonful of each portion of food on the plate to help empower you around food.
So this is responding to physical hunger by tuning into your stomach and taste buds by asking yourself – What would I like to eat now? And allowing yourself to eat whatever you want until physically full.
Likewise, respond to emotional hunger by tuning into your emotions and feelings. Name the feeling and emotional issue if possible. Ask yourself – Given the fact I feel this way what would I like to do now? And follow up on the appropriate, healthy answer.
Respond to physical fullness by not eating until physically hungry again.

## Guideline 2

Raising self-acceptance. When we raise our self-acceptance, what in fact, we are saying is – I take responsibility for my size, shape and eating habits. Through acceptance we start to make the shift from blaming our fat for our problems to taking responsibility for finding real solutions to those problems. No more are we thinking – 'If only I was slim that would not have happened.' We realise that slimness in itself does not solve our problems. Being slim in itself does not change our lives. Positive ideas and positive action does.

We are owing our fat by accepting it, and remember – we have to own something before we can lose it. This is just as true of excess weight as it is of anything else we might lose. Therefore, by increasing our self-acceptance and really feeling a positive sense of owning our excess weight, we are putting ourselves in the position to lose that excess weight once and for all.

No longer judging our excess weight, no longer denying its existence, no longer condemning it as repulsive, but rather we begin to see it as it is, in a non-judgemental light. It is, after all, the result of us having used food when full to stuff down our feelings. Uncomfortable feelings and the subconscious desire to suppress them caused us to crave food when we were not even physically hungry. Giving in to that craving, we ate when we were physically full and that is what caused the excess weight. Excess eating (eating when physically full) causes excess weight. This is the cycle of addiction.

Important note: It is not the type of foods we eat (so called fattening foods) that makes us fat. It is eating when we are already physically full that causes us to gain weight.

So, cease the self-criticism and blame. After all you would not beat up on a recovering alcoholic or drug addict. You would have some respect for the enormity of the task she is undertaking. Be that forgiving and understanding of yourself. Be that accepting of yourself. Food addiction is just as tricky to overcome as any other addiction and you deserve encouragement, help, understanding and respect, both from deep within yourself and from others.

In general, if we have a problem with weight, eating and food, we do not know how to experience certain feelings comfortably, so we stuff them down with food. Stuffing feelings down with food is one way of dealing with them and by no means the only way. It deals with feelings by suppressing them rather than resolving them. Suppressing our feelings with food is not a great idea, mainly because it causes us to eat regardless of whether we are physically hungry or not, causes us to gain weight and gives us an eating disorder.

Now, as we learn how to break out of those negative eating patterns and find new alternative ways of dealing with our feelings (ways that involve resolving feelings rather than suppressing them) we allow ourselves, not only to alter the way we eat, but we also enable ourselves to heal that eating disorder, and lose any excess weight that has been gained as a result of those old eating habits.

## That precious inner seed

Self-acceptance is like a precious inner seed which can be nurtured, tended and allowed to grow, blossom and bear the fabulous fruits of self-confidence, self-esteem and self-worth. Contrary to popular belief, self-acceptance does not magically appear when one is slim. This is because it is not an attribute of slimness. It is not some positive trait, that we are guaranteed, solely as a result of our becoming slim. It is not something slim people have and fat people do not have. Self-acceptance is not automatically part and parcel of being a slim person for there are many slim people without self-acceptance. It is not inexorably linked with being slim. It is not the package deal that the media, diet and fashion industry constantly bombards us with.

**Popular myth:** Slimness alone guarantees self-acceptance, confidence and self-assurance.

Your self-acceptance is not an outcome of how fat or slim you are now. Self-acceptance develops within us in childhood as a direct result of good, loving, acceptance-filled parenting. If you have low self-acceptance it can be attributed to how you were treated as a child and the conclusions you made about that treatment. Lack of parental approval, lack of emotional support. Physical, sexual or psychological abuse are some of the contributing factors towards low self-acceptance that a child could carry into adulthood.

High self-acceptance is even more than a frame of mind, it is a state of awareness, it is a conscious and subconscious belief system that can only be attained by doing emotional work on yourself through affirmation, therapy, self-help books and the like. It does indeed need to be consciously cultivated.

If you do not accept yourself now at the larger size, it is a sure sign of a belief system containing thoughts of a self-critical nature – the opposite of self-acceptance. If you had negative, critical, emotionally distant or otherwise abusive parents it is no surprise that your subconscious thoughts and beliefs systems would be of low self-acceptance. Or that you turn to food when full to alleviate the painful feelings associated with a dysfunctional upbringing. (By belief system I mean thoughts and opinions that you believe to be true).

If we have low self-acceptance when fat, we will not be able to accept ourselves at a smaller size either unless we do the emotional work required to change our negative thoughts and belief systems into self-accepting ones.

**Your point of power is in the ever present now!** You can raise your self-acceptance now regardless of the past and regardless of your present size. It is worth all the effort, allowing that inner seed of self-acceptance to be actively nurtured and encouraged to grow. Believe me, if you have low self-acceptance at your larger size, when you get slim, your self-acceptance will stay at the exact same critically low level until you do something to raise it.

You may still think your self-acceptance depends on your weight, and that once you get slim you will automatically be more accepting of yourself. The truth is however, with low self-acceptance, no matter how slim you are, you can always find something to criticise!

So, with the resolve to do the emotional work to raise self-acceptance, the tools that are mentioned later are the means by which we can do just that. Practised on a daily basis, self-acceptance can reach new heights! By accepting ourselves, our size and shape we are not only becoming more responsible, self-acceptance encourages a greater self-awareness and a knowing of how all is connected. Our feelings and how we deal with them, is connected to how we eat; and how we eat effects our weight. Our unresolved emotional issues and feelings, and the need to suppress or avoid them, causes us to crave food when we are in fact physically full. Giving in to this craving by eating when full, not only suppresses our feelings but also saps our energy and causes weight gain.

Heightened awareness of ourselves and our eating patterns, acknowledges, that the excess weight got there by completely overriding the sensations of being physically hungry and (more specifically) being physically full until they were meaningless strangers rather than loving guides.

So, as we start to look at our own bodies without judgement or criticism, let's read on, and discover exactly how our size and shape alters and changes naturally as a result of following our three guidelines. Let's explore how we can practice the guidelines until they are all working together in harmony, producing the result of a slim body and a healthy, non-addicted relationship to food.

The goal of self-acceptance is to be able to say – *Yes, I accept myself, my size and shape unconditionally now* – and believe it. How can this be achieved? The simplest way is to get into the habit of writing out affirmations and repeating them silently in your mind for at least five minutes a day, every day. Try the above statement in italics. It is an excellent affirmation. As you are affirming it, notice how you feel, notice the thoughts that come to mind. Do these thoughts agree or disagree with the affirmation? You probably will not believe the affirmation at first. Don't worry about this, just keep on repeating it until you do. (We may be talking about a few days work, or this might take daily work for about a month or more).

Find reasons to believe the positive affirmation. Be aware of your thoughts of disbelief and wave them goodbye. You can surround them with a pink bubble and see them float away, for these negative thoughts are even now being replaced by the delightfully positive and nurturing idea of self-acceptance through the persistent repetition of the healing affirmation – I accept myself, my size and shape unconditionally now.

> Self-acceptance and positive change go hand in hand.
> Self-criticism gives negative habits the power to repeat themselves.

**Written work**: List, with a pen and paper, three or more reasons why you do not accept your size and shape unconditionally right now. Then tear up this list, burn it or flush it down the toilet to symbolise the fact that you are dissolving these negative thoughts and ideas. Then list three or more reasons why you can and should accept your size and shape unconditionally right now. Keep this list. Carry it with you in your wallet or handbag and look at it often. Repeat those positive statements as new affirmations. Say them aloud in private, write them out repeatedly and consciously think them whenever you feel the need to remind yourself of why you can and should accept yourself unconditionally right now.

## More about self-acceptance

Most women resist this idea of self-acceptance because they feel that by accepting their size and shape they are giving up all hope of ever changing it. In fact the exact opposite is true. Self-acceptance is a necessary prerequisite to natural, permanent, weight loss and true happiness with that result.

Remember: Self-acceptance, truly means accepting ourselves as we are, before we get slim, whilst saying 'NO' to a future of excess weight by healing our addiction to food when full.

## Self-acceptance gives us our accurate starting point

When we know and accept where we are, we can then accurately plan our route to where we want to go. Where we are now is our present weight, eating patterns and emotional baggage. Where we want to go is our slim self, a healthy relationship to food and the ability to resolve our emotional issues as opposed to suppressing them by eating when full. Using the tools in this book you are now able to plot your own accurate course towards that desired destination.

The self-accepting attitude says without judgement – This is me. I am this size and shape. I have this weight problem / eating disorder. I accept that I have this problem at this present moment in my life. I also accept that I do not want this problem in my life. I am not in denial about it, in fact I am actively working on healing it and I accept full responsibility for healing it.

This kind of self-acceptance is very empowering and necessary in the process of healing an eating disorder. Hence, the self-accepting, non-judgemental attitude, actually puts us in the position where we are no longer in denial of our problem but can move forward and tackle that problem more effectively, thus helping us lose our excess weight for good.

You can affirm – 'Yes, I accept my size and shape as it is now. I also accept the fact that my size and shape alters and changes as I alter and change my eating habits. I now take responsibility for altering and changing my eating habits and as I eat when hungry and stop when full I am enabling my body to establish its own perfect weight permanently and naturally.'

Through self-acceptance we are not only taking responsibility for our size and shape, we are also accepting and taking responsibility for the fact that our excess weight got there by us eating when we were physically full. We were either consciously or subconsciously trying to deal with our feelings by stuffing them down with food when full. Now, rather than obsessing about our body and food, we can be focused on losing any excess weight permanently through allowing our relationship to food become a healthy non-addicted one by following our three main guidelines, mentioned previously, and explained fully throughout this book. What we are gaining is a new and strengthened understanding!

**Some effective tools for raising self-acceptance**

1.      Look in the mirror, keeping eye contact with yourself repeat this affirmation silently in your mind at least 15 times: (Your name) I love you, approve of you and accept you unconditionally now. Do this exercise as often as possible, ideally once in the morning and once at night, every day until you feel you believe those words.

2.      Make a habit of looking at yourself in a full length mirror without judging your reflection. If necessary view yourself as you would a work of art that you do not really like but are trying hard to appreciate. Notice where you curve in and out. Notice how clothes look on you. Notice your skin tones and cast out that inner judge. Replace her with a loving, accepting, wise inner friend. Just accept your reflection – no story about it, no judgments about it. It is what it is, and it deserves acceptance and love. Do this regularly until you feel the acceptance begin to flow and every time you look in the mirror you can find acceptance and appreciation looking back at you.

Written affirmations are of course wonderful and very effective for changing our negative thought patterns and belief systems. With self-acceptance our task is to change the – I do not accept my size and shape – thought pattern, to the all-encompassing – I accept myself, my size and shape now – thought pattern. This is the thought pattern that you presume will automatically appear when you are slim and I say: 'If you work at raising your self-acceptance to this high level now, then, you will have the opportunity to take it with you when you get slim. In fact it will automatically do so.'

Your subconscious belief systems and thoughts are like a filter through which you view yourself and the world. In fact they are not only a filter but they greatly influence and indeed create the life you see before you. They can affect the experiences in your day to day living. Therefore it is very useful to practice affirmations daily as they enable the development of a conscious awareness of previously subconscious negative beliefs. It is like the positive affirmation wakes up the negative beliefs you have about yourself and thus you become aware of them; and once aware of them you can replace them with positive, life-affirming, slim-friendly thoughts and beliefs through continued repetition of your chosen affirmations. Thus you are working on changing and healing at the very source of your problems – Your own negative thoughts and beliefs.

Through affirmations, this bringing up, clearing and changing process causes the new positive thought to become a permanent, positive belief system that actually helps you change into healthier eating habits. You believe it to be true. You feel it is true. This positive self-accepting belief system firmly planted in the subconscious spawns positive spin-offs such as high self-esteem, a sense of security and confidence in one's self and one's ability. Not forgetting increased power to being positive change into one's own life.

## A few words about birth

I personally believe that we are conscious entities from the moment we are conceived, also how we are treated as new born babies needs to be especially gentle, loving and safe in order for us to have a positive impression about life. In other words the thought we had as we took our first breath formed a cellular blueprint upon which our whole life gets based. Conclusions such as 'Nobody loves me. I can't get what I want. Life is painful. People hurt me. I don't want to be here,' are common conclusions many of us made upon birth. Reading 'Birth Without Violence' by Dr Fredrick LeBoyer really helps clarify what I am saying here.

However, unless you do rebirthing breathwork or deep meditation you are not likely to remember what you concluded on taking your first breath, and although it can be helpful, if you are not drawn to do that, then it is not necessary; because often as you are repeating a positive affirmation you may realise other, more recent sources of where your negative thoughts came from – a scolding parent or teacher perhaps, a sibling or a bully at school. It is good to just notice any unhappy memories and know that they have no power over you now, as you are discharging the energy of them through simply being aware of them and feeling the feelings associated with them. Feelings are like clouds in the sky – They pass! We no longer have to suppress them. We just need to feel and heal. And that comes through awareness.

Just as negative thoughts can be turned into their positive opposites, negative memories can be re-worked. After you remember a painful incident from your past, take a moment to re-live it, uncomfortable though it may be. Recall those present, what was said and done, shed tears if sadness comes up, beat pillows if anger arises. Affirm when you feel ready – This is finished, this is over, I declare it and any negative effects of this erased forever through the power of (….) fill in whatever you consider a power divine. Now visualise what you would have liked to have happen instead. This is re-working an old memory. Now in this healing you may decide to never see those who inflicted pain on you again. Reworking an old memory does <u>not</u> mean that all is well and you can open yourself up to abuse again. It instead strengthens your ability to create healthy boundaries between yourself and people who have caused you or your loved ones harm in the past. If they are not already out of your life then maybe it is time to protect yourself from them by never seeing them again, be they a family member, a friend, co-worker or boss.

**Example of a negative belief:** You may find yourself at work, frustrated because you are finding it impossible to meet a certain deadline. You find the thought 'I am not good enough' flash across your mind. Say a mental 'No' to this thought and consciously change it to 'I am good enough. I am good enough. I am good enough.' At such times it is doubly reinforcing to remind yourself of your accomplishments and successes of the past no matter how small.

Likewise, if on your way home you catch a glimpse of yourself in a shop window and think – 'I look awful today' – mentally say – 'No, I look fine today.' You might also add – 'I must get a haircut or get a new coat or tackle my financial problems.' That is okay. This is not about being in denial about your appearance or problems. It is also, not about beating yourself up about your appearance or problems. It is about taking responsibility for your appearance and problems in a non-judgmental, positive way. Affirming you are fine the way you are, whilst acknowledging that you are also willing to work on changing whatever you wish to change, is empowering. Take whatever steps you can to bring about the changes you want and be an encouragement to yourself rather than a harsh critic.

As you continue to affirm and re-affirm your unconditional self-acceptance you are developing a very healthy attitude indeed. Just have fun being positive about yourself. In this way you are truly nurturing yourself with compliments and gentle praise, sure forerunners of wellbeing.

Believing and feeling, that we do completely accept our size and shape, is such an essential part of losing excess weight this way, that it is one of the major keys. Just as you cannot open a locked door without a key, to attempt permanent weight loss and happiness with that result, without this important key, is just as unrealistic. Needless to say, the time and effort put into developing self-acceptance is rewarded a thousand times over. Increased peace of mind and calmness. Self-confidence and self-worth built on a solid foundation. A heightened sense of integrity, security and a positive sense of self, all emerge as a result of allowing the seed of self-acceptance to grow.

The inner garden is a Garden of Eden. Learning to let it blossom and flourish is a skill we can all acquire with patience and knowledge. Thought is creative. With an inner Garden of Eden, imagine how the outer world, which is it's reflection, looks.

**A few things to remember about self-acceptance**
1. It does not mean we have to stay the same weight.
2. It actually puts us in the position from which we are able to lose any excess weight permanently and feel happy with that result.
3. It is about taking responsibility.
4. It is about acknowledging rather than judging.
5. It is the first step towards liking ourselves and having a healthy self-love.
6. It is empowering.

7.     It is about taking the pressure off and lightening up by saying – This is me and I am okay.
8.     It is facing up to the truth about yourself with kindness, forgiveness, love and understanding.
9.     It is the seed that blossoms into self-confidence, self-esteem, self-worth, security and assertiveness.
10.    It is the first step in becoming the person you want to be.

## Guideline 3

<u>Pinpointing and resolving emotional issues rather than suppressing them.</u> This is relatively easy when you remember to ask yourself - What feeling is this? And – Given the fact I feel this way, what would I like to do now? The answers are all within you. By asking those two questions you can access those answers. Thus, finding the alternatives to stuffing down feelings! Yes, the answers to those questions provides us with the alternative way of dealing with our previously unresolved (suppressed) emotional issues and feelings. Thus enabling us to pinpoint and resolve our feelings and emotional issues rather than stuffing them down with food eaten when full.

Question: What if I cannot get in contact with my feelings? What if, they stay 'stuffed down' (suppressed)?

Answer: We can all get in contact with the feelings we have previously suppressed and I will show you how. Firstly, wait for a moment in the day when you feel like eating but you are already physically full. Secondly, say to yourself: I know I am physically full. Now what feeling or emotion is this? What words can best describe the way I feel emotionally? Is this feeling located in any particular area of my body and what sort of sensation it? (Such as butterflies in my stomach or a tightness in my throat?) The answer to these questions will put you in contact with your feelings. It is possible that you are not able to put into words what you are feeling and that is fine. Description is not essential. It is enough just to feel the feelings and notice the energy in your body. Thirdly, practice, practice and then practice some more!

**Healthy Options**
It is useful to make a list of all the things you enjoy. List as many activities as you can, such as walking in the park, having a coffee and chat with a friend, swimming. Also include new activities you would like to try, such as learning a foreign language, or attending an art course at your local college. So, if you get stuck for answers when you ask yourself – Given the fact I feel this way, what would I like to do now? You can consult your list of enjoyable activities to help prompt you into action.

Most of you are already, pretty much aware of what your own personal emotional issues are. It could be boredom, anger, sadness, depression, pain or frustration, which you try to alleviate with food. Your unresolved emotional issues could be about a failed relationship, poverty, an unhappy childhood, inadequate living conditions, career choices or even birth trauma.

**To heal and resolve whatever your issues may be:**
Firstly requires awareness of which particular feelings and emotional issues, send you, when physically full, to the refrigerator or biscuit tin without so much as a backward glance.
Secondly allow yourself to <u>not eat when physically full</u> and feel these emotions.
Thirdly find and practice, practical and workable ways to deal with these, your own personal emotional issues and dilemmas.
Finally you will know that you have resolved an emotional issue when you can think or talk about that issue, that used to cause you pain, and you realise the pain has gone. Freedom indeed!

**Comfort Eating**
We have all heard of comfort eating. We know that we are trying to get comfort and emotional satisfaction, from food alone, anytime we catch ourselves eating when we are not, in truth, physically hungry. What would truly give us emotional peace of mind is something much more complicated than fixing ourselves a sandwich when we are not even physically hungry.
Resolving our emotional issues requires that we actively put into practice the answer that we get when we ask ourselves the key question: Given the fact I feel this way, what would I like to do now? Putting into practice the answer to this question enables us to resolve the issue we are dealing with. It may be guidance to read a certain book, say some affirmations or listen to some calming music, phone a friend, go for a walk or take a course. Whatever the answer is, as long as it is a healthy one, follow it

up, even if you feel a bit scared. In fact, expect to feel scared, as this is almost certain to bring up your fears. You are learning how to deal with fear too, you know!

## Food Pleasure not Suppression Pressure

Food, what is in fact the source of nutritional sustenance, can also be the source of very pleasurable sensations in terms of taste and the ease of healthy digestion. It is a satisfying, nurturing experience to eat when one is physically hungry and to satisfy that hunger by eating, what one truly fancies eating at that moment in time and stopping when full. This is completely different to the forced, abusive sense of comfort one tries to attain from eating food when one is already physically full.

So, as you can see, if you are using food to stuff down your anger, boredom, depression etc. the next logical step is to address these feelings and emotional issues and deal with them in more effective ways. In other words, learn to acknowledge how you feel, ask yourself – 'What's the solution? How can I move forward? What's the healthy alternative to suppressing this issue? What would I like to do now?' Follow up on the healthy guidance, that inner answer, and thus you are helping yourself resolve your previously unresolved emotional issues. Once your emotional issues are resolved, a more natural, pleasurable and healthy relationship to food is allowed to evolve. Food is no longer used to suppress feelings. It is no longer the object of your addiction. In fact, you even cease craving food to suppress your feelings and emotional issues once they have already been resolved.

Loving food does not mean we have to be overweight. Being slim does not mean that we have to deny ourselves our favourite foods. When we overcome compulsive eating, food really does become a pleasure.

**What is the difference between my fat self and my thin self?**
List all the things that you think would be different if you were slim.
For example:
1. I would be more attractive.
2. My clothes would fit better.
3. I would attract a soul mate / partner more easily.

Now, here's the tricky bit – write down the various ways you could achieve that same result but without getting slim.
For example:
1. How I would be more attractive without getting slim.

Well, I can pay more attention to the clothes I wear and experiment with different styles of dress and make up, just for fun.

I also resolve to cease criticising the way I look, and instead I will find something to praise in my appearance. That way I am sure to feel more attractive and if I feel attractive I will look attractive.

I can begin to see my attractiveness. I can affirm daily – 'My name, I believe you are an attractive woman!' - whilst keeping eye contact with myself in the mirror. I can persist with this until I believe it.

By keeping eye contact with yourself, you are starting with the attractiveness in your eyes and everyone has attractive eyes, especially when self-acceptance and love shine through them. Another good affirmation is: <u>Every day in every way I am experiencing natural beauty, light and life.</u> What an attractive thought to have in your subconscious. A thought that can surely bring about attractive results!

2.      How clothes can fit better without getting slim.

I shall buy myself clothes that fit me now at this size, in the styles I really like. I could buy elasticised waists in my skirts so I can feel more comfortable and will fit perfectly.

I will get that suit altered so that it fits me now, at the size I am now.

3.      How I can attract a partner without getting slim.

I could write out a list of the qualities I want in my ideal partner. I can visualise myself going out on a date and enjoying an evening with an interesting man. Thus psychologically preparing myself for a successful, delightful date. I can work on dissolving any fears I might have around having a relationship and intimacy.

I can get out and participate in activities I enjoy. Thus giving myself the chance to meet a partner who has the same interests as me.

I could think about how people in general attract and repel each other. What subtle signals are given and received. I could analyse the signals I send out and consider if they are appropriate.

Look closely at the various ways you can achieve your desired result, without having to wait until you are slim. Choose the ideas that appeal to you the most and start to incorporate them into your daily life as much as possible so you can get valuable feedback or good results. This way you can achieve those desired states first listed, through looking at and doing what it really takes to achieve them, rather than assuming that all this happens just as a result of being slim. You will also be achieving your slim figure by eating when physically hungry and stopping when physically full.

Just like following up on the healthy answers to our important question – 'Given the fact I feel this way, what would I like to do now?' – the incorporation into your day to day life, of activities like in the aforementioned examples, is very important. For this is the practical work that gets you your own personal results. So take action! Appropriate action! The more you actually do those activities, the richer your life will become as you realise that the things you want in life do not come as a result of being slim alone, but rather as a result of you personally making the effort and taking those necessary and sometimes scary steps, towards their achievement.

## You will become slim

As I have already mentioned, you will become slim as a result of eating when you are physically hungry and stopping when you are physically full. To stop eating when physically full is made easier and indeed possible when you are appropriately addressing your own emotional issues. Instead of using food when full to deal with your emotional hunger you are acknowledging how you feel, asking yourself what you would like to do and following up on the healthy answer. Thus you are nurturing yourself emotionally, feeding yourself emotionally in these new, healthy and truly satisfying ways. You can see now that this is a two pronged attack on the compulsive behaviour:

1.  You are relating to your physical hunger appropriately by eating when physically hungry and stopping when physically full.
2.  You are relating to your emotional needs appropriately by actually addressing the emotional issue rather than suppressing it.

With all this appropriate activity there is no room for addicted activity! Thus you break free from addiction and knock this complex phenomenon called food addiction well and truly on the head, seeing it for what it is, an in-adequate means of dealing with feelings and emotional issues. It now lies dead, like the discarded habit it is. No longer a threat, but simply something you understand and have no use for, having replaced it with good health, psychological and physical strength, personal achievement and fulfilment.

## The Adventure Begins!

This journey is a joyous one, of self-discovery, support, friendship making, increased love and respect for one's own body, and the awakening of something we thought we had lost, but instead had only temporarily forgotten – how to listen to ourselves, our needs and respond accordingly. It is an experimentation of what we can do, and a discovery of what brings us joy. It is a lightening up process, from within out, both physically and psychologically. It is the only road to be on. The road of personal expansion and growth. Effortless expansion into the good that we desire and the life that we want. This road leads us right into an improved life. No longer expanding our body size by using food to suppress our feelings, we are instead, expanding our very selves into the joy of life. Joy that comes from working towards and achieving your own heart-felt desires in each area of your life including career, relationships, finances and health. As we grow, harmony replaces disharmony, love replaces fear. Courage and strength coexist and all our efforts and rewards are equally balanced.

A new, truer way of being evolves and flourishes as we each fulfil our own unique potential, in all areas of life. This is the alternative to stuffing down our feelings. This is being alive! This is the experience of feeling our feelings!

## Slim and healthy

It is wise to want to be slim and healthy. To be slim and healthy is a goal all of us can certainly achieve. Being obsessed with food and weight is, however, a very different story. Obsessive behaviour has its roots firmly planted in the fertile soil of unresolved emotional issues, suppressed feelings and ideas of lack and limitation. How we deal with our unresolved emotional issues and problems is an important factor in contributing to how healthy we are.

Let's go back to basics. An unresolved emotional issue is simply something we have not let learned:

(a)     How to deal with in such a way, that we can change it into something more favourable to us.

Or

(b)     How to change our perspective on it, so that we feel more comfortable and accepting of it.

In fact, often when we change our perspective on a problem, we often open the way for the perfect solution to appear. When we eat beyond physical fullness we block that way. We stuff down or suppress the problem and our feelings about it rather than deal with it in a more appropriate way. However, now that we are healing our eating habit, one of our main goals is to find that more appropriate way. We focus on discovering practical, workable solutions to our day to day problems and emotional issues. We learn how to feel more comfortable with ourselves and our feelings. As we cease avoiding our feelings, and as we find ways to deal with our emotional issues, we are no longer turning to food in order to stuff those feelings down.

Any time we find ourselves – Not physically hungry but still wanting to eat – is a good time to check in with our feelings. This eating when we are already physically full, is, eating that is done in order to stuff down or suppress a feeling or emotional issue. Sometimes we are not aware of the emotional issue or feeling. We are only aware of the need to binge, or eat those ten extra biscuits when already definitely, physically full, and we end up wondering - 'Why am I eating this, I am not even hungry?'

Eating until you experience an uncomfortable overfullness in your stomach could be your normal eating pattern. This is the pattern that you can alter and change to – eating when physically hungry and stopping when physically full.

As I have already mentioned, this stuffing down of an emotional issue (which occurs when we eat even though the stomach is physically full) is the same as suppressing it. Anytime you find yourself eating even though you feel physically full, know that you are eating to suppress some feeling or emotional issue. Why else would you want to eat when your stomach is already physically full and busily digesting its contents? Physically you do not require that food. Your stomach is full. It is uncomfortable to overeat and uncomfortable to carry around the excess weight. So why do you do this? The answer is sure and simple. You do this in order to stuff down (suppress) the feelings and emotional issues, that you have not yet learned, how to deal with in a healthier way.

In order to suppress an emotional issue or feeling you must do something, that something is addiction. Therefore this eating when already physically full is a sign of addiction, and an activity of addiction. So, let's not underestimate the enormity of our task here. It is no longer a matter of just counting calories, getting slim and suddenly all of your life is perfect. No, it goes a little deeper than that. What we are, in fact, doing is giving up an addiction – an addiction to food when full.

Remember, any activity that is done in order to suppress an emotional issue or feeling is, addiction. <u>And the first step we take, to break the cycle of addiction is, simply, to get in touch with the feelings and emotional issues which we have previously been spending a lot of time and energy suppressing or stuffing down with food.</u> Once we allow ourselves to experience these feelings and emotional issues we are well on the way to resolving them. It is good to know that when we are busily experiencing our feelings, we can be certain that we are not suppressing them. For, experiencing a feeling or emotional issue, is the opposite of suppressing it.

## What is suppression?

Suppression is one way of dealing with an unresolved emotional issue or feeling with which we may be uncomfortable. It involves putting feelings and emotional issues below our level of awareness, into the subconscious. This takes a lot of energy. Suppression loses its appeal when we find a more appropriate and altogether joyous way of dealing with those same feelings and emotional issues.

Let's get clear about suppression. It serves a purpose. It is a learned habit, and this is one habit that can be changed, if we want to take the time, follow the appropriate steps and are willing to feel our feelings.

Uncomfortable with a feeling, we deal with it in what may be the only way we know how, by suppressing it. However, in order to resolve our emotional issues, it is necessary that we feel our feelings. If these feelings are of a very intense nature, possibly associated with some past trauma, then feeling those feelings is not the easiest thing in the world to do! It takes the terror out of confronting traumatic emotional issues if you know that you can deal with the intensity of these emotions and feelings. There is no feeling that cannot be felt, or has not been felt, experienced and overcome by someone else before you. Feeling a feeling allows it to integrate, and once integrated, the trauma is over. One is at peace. Healed - if you like.

It is the suppression of feeling that causes us trouble in the form of addiction, ill health, financial or relationship problems. There are great advantages in being courageous and feeling the unpleasant feelings of the past and present. Going through the experience of discomfort in order to experience the benefits in terms of inner peace, health, personal and professional fulfilment make it all worthwhile. In my opinion one of the most effective methods for accessing and dealing with big emotional issues is a breathing technique called - Rebirthing.

Through feeling your feelings and working on your own personal growth you can still be the person you would have been, had you had the most loving, healthy, supportive and emotionally present parents in the world. This is because your power lies in the conclusions you make and the healing you have through integrating the trauma. It is healing what happened to you, as opposed to suppressing what happened to you.

For example: A person could have had a relatively good upbringing but made negative conclusions about it and thus suffer as a result of those negative conclusions. Likewise, a person could have had a lot of trauma and challenges in her upbringing but learns how to deal with them constructively, seeks healing and makes positive conclusions - such as: 'Well, I must have paid off a huge karmic debt!' Or – 'In facing and overcoming the past I am able to show others that trauma need not kill you or cause you to be an addict or overweight.' Thus emerging the victor of those past experiences.

## The path of integration

Step 1. Being aware of when you are suppressing your feelings. As regards to compulsive eating, this is becoming aware of what you are doing anytime you are eating even though you are physically full. You become a non-judgmental observer of your own compulsive behaviour.

Step 2. Being willing to stop that behaviour which enables you to suppress your feelings. In other words, you are willing to try to stop eating when physically full. You can do this by cutting through and arresting the compulsion with the thought – What feeling is this? What feeling is this? Keep repeating this question silently until you become aware of the feelings, and, at times you can even stop that binge.

Step 3. Actually stop eating when physically full. While no longer eating when physically full, being open to experiencing emotions that may feel a bit uncomfortable.

Step 4. Whilst experiencing your emotions, being open and willing to find healthy ways of dealing with those emotions and emotional issues by asking yourself the question – Given the fact I feel this way, what would I like to do now?

Step 5. Listening to your inner guidance, those inner whisperings that are answering that question.

Once you have turned your ear inwards, listened for and received your answer, you check up on that answer, obviously making sure it is legal, healthy and does not harm yourself or another. Thereby, insuring that it is a healthy way to deal with your emotions, which does not involve further suppression of these emotions.

Step 6. Get busy doing it! Follow that inner guidance! Act on that healthy answer! Allow it to lead you out of your addictions and into a slim, healthy, addiction-free life.

**The healthy answer**

You may say – How am I supposed to know this healthy, appropriate way of dealing with my feelings and emotional issues? Well, the answer is simple. If there is a compulsive feel to anything you do, or think about doing, simply relax and see if you can stay with your feelings. Healthy answers usually have a relaxed and somewhat joyous quality to them. Be wary of a compulsive jog, or shopping spree that has no joy. Cigarettes, alcohol and drugs are obvious substances that one needs to check for compulsive urges towards. Staying with your feelings as much as you can while continuing to ask yourself the question – Given the fact I feel this way, what would I like to do now? – will bring you to a healthy answer that you will recognise sooner or later.

I feel it is of the utmost importance for you to be supported at this time. So ask yourself – Who is supporting me through this? Unless you have an answer to this one, see about getting some support, be it professional help or just a friend with whom to say affirmations or do healing visualisations.

Further awareness can be gained by tuning in to your feelings and asking yourself: What is this feeling trying to tell me? Really listen to your thoughts and intuitive whispers coming from your higher self.

This is subtle inner work and it takes practice to master. Through turning your attention inward you can quickly discover what is the best course of action to take at any given moment in time. If you allow yourself to recognise and trust this inner guidance, you can be accurately guided to the perfect solution by your gut feelings, common sense and intuition. The answers are all within you and by asking the appropriate questions such as the ones already mentioned you can access these priceless answers.

## Our relationship to food

A woman with an eating disorder can have such a warped relationship to food that she overrides the subtle inner cues which are telling her whether her stomach is full or empty. She can be so out of touch with when she is physically hungry and when she is physically full that she is stuffing her face when her stomach is screaming at her - No more food please!! And when her stomach is saying: I would like a nice hot bowl of soup. She refuses to eat. This is an example of a woman not meeting her needs appropriately. She is indulging in this self-abusive activity in order to suppress her feelings. This is, as I have mentioned before, one way of dealing with unpleasant feelings and unresolved emotional issues. Whatever these feelings or issues may be, she is using food to suppress them. Is that woman you?

Question: So how do we begin to break out of this inappropriate cycle, which is a very self-abusive way of dealing with feelings and emotional issues?

Answer: We learn the difference between physical hunger and emotional hunger.

We acknowledge that what is actually happening to us when we crave food, even though our stomachs are physically full, is the tendency towards addiction kicking in. To put it another way, the craving to eat when physically full, is the compulsive urge to suppress our feelings due to the fact that we simply have not yet learned any other way of dealing with those feelings.

We ask ourselves – 'What is the healthy alternative to stuffing my feelings down?' Or, our old reliable - 'What feeling is this? And given the fact I feel this way what would I like to do now?' We practice that healthy, alternative way of dealing with our feelings.

The following shows us how to do just that! Practice asking yourself often the key question – Am I physically hungry? And following through on the guidelines in columns A and B of this all important process – The Am I Hungry? Process. The first few weeks and months of healing you eating habit can be spent mastering this simple, empowering procedure. Anytime you think about food or eating ask yourself – Am I Hungry?

(A)

Am I physically hungry?

If the answer is 'Yes' then:

Eat whatever you fancy until physically full. When physically full stop eating until physically hungry again.

(B)

Am I physically hungry?

If the answer is 'No' then:

This is emotional hunger, when you still want to eat even though you are physically full. In this instant it is important to ask yourself the following:

1. What feeling is this?

2.　　Given the fact I feel this way, what would I like to do now?

3.　　If the answer is a healthy one then get busy doing it!

Do be aware of what your mind comes up with as an answer to the question – Given the fact I feel this way, what would I like to do now? Make sure the answer is the healthy alternative to stuffing the feelings down, and not just another avoidance tactic. It is important to allow yourself to feel your feelings. It is also important that how you act on them is helping you resolve them.

**Definition of emotional hunger** – Feeling 'hungry' and wanting to eat when your stomach is actually physically full. Your stomach is already physically full of food and in the process of digesting that food. Feeling hungry in the mouth as opposed to the stomach. This is a compulsion to eat when full. A craving to eat when full, and it is a mainly subconscious urge to run away from how you are feeling emotionally. Eating when full puts uncomfortable emotions into suppression, that is, below your level of awareness.

**Definition of physical hunger** – Feeling hungry, wanting to eat when actually physically hungry. Your stomach is empty or partially empty and it is both essential and healthy to eat at this time, for this hunger is the natural, healthy desire to feed and nourish the body appropriately in order to stay alive.

Example: You feel like eating and you check in with your stomach. You ask yourself: (1) Am I physically hungry? The answer comes 'No I am physically full.' Your stomach feels full and you know you have just 5 mins before finished quite a big meal. (2) What feeling is this? And you realise you are bored. You then ask yourself. (3) Given the fact I feel this way, what would I like to do now? The answer comes, I would like to phone a friend. You get your phone and call one of your friends, enjoy a chat and feel satisfied.

This is a simple example of easily meeting your own emotional needs appropriately. Needs that had the potential to cause you to overeat. I do not have to remind you that it is not always as simple as this. There could be bigger issues involved. The important thing is to become aware of those issues, feel the feelings associated with those issues and know deep within you lies the solution to those issues no matter how old or painful they may be. Thus you face up to and resolve them, leaving you free to move forward into a life of your choice not burdened by the habit of eating when full and excess weight.

Whilst in the process of changing our unhealthy eating patterns, the more we are able to recognise and act appropriately on emotional hunger and physical hunger, the easier it is to get into contact with the previously suppressed emotional issues and feelings. The more we eat when physically hungry and stop when physically full, the more we experience those old suppressed feelings. The more we get used to experiencing our feelings, the less scared we are of them. We can then discover what they are all about and go about resolving them effectively and permanently.

Once resolved, these emotional issues and feelings, never again cause us to eat when we are physically full in order to cope with them. Now, we are in the powerful position of not only being able to cope with our feelings and emotional issues but we are also well on the way to resolving permanently anything that previously troubled us.

### Choice (A) The self-abusive 'stuff feelings down' way

You have your emotional issue and uncomfortable feelings – you suppress your feelings. This involves indulging in your addiction (eating when full) thus depleting or blocking your vital life force energy or chi. This energy is so subtle you won't physically notice it, but nevertheless you are suppressing it and your feelings by eating even though you are, in truth, already physically full. Or, you may start off hungry, eat until full but continue to eat long past physical fullness.

### Choice (B) The healthy 'feel feelings' way

You have your emotional issue and uncomfortable feelings – you experience your feelings thus helping them integrate, and you think about the solution to the emotional issue thus helping resolve it. This involves eating if you are physically hungry, not eating if you are physically full. Naming your feelings and what they are about, anger, fear, grief, boredom etc then asking yourself our much-repeated valuable question: Given the fact I feel this way what would I like to do now? Ask this whenever you are already physically full but still crave to eat more, for it will always guide you away from your addiction and towards good health and a healed relationship to food.

The use of the tools, suggestions and concepts throughout this book along with you yourself finding and using your own healthy appropriate ways of dealing with your feelings are major keys to natural permanent weight loss.

So now, at this point in your life, as you are willing to approach weight loss from a perspective of unravelling the deeper causes of your excess weight and eating habits, let's explore together, step by step, in detail, how you either suppress or integrate your feelings.

First you become aware of what you are doing, that is, you become aware of when you are doing something to suppress your feelings and then gradually try to bring in the healthy alternative. The repeated use of the healthy alternative to stuffing your feelings down, becomes, your normal way of dealing with feelings and emotional issues that arise in your daily life.

Integrating your feelings instead of suppressing them is very energising and a great relief. Asking yourself – Am I hungry? – to get in tune with the bodily sensations of hunger and fullness is the natural way to permanent weight loss and establishing your own natural weight effortlessly.

Knowing when we are using food to stuff feelings down and practicing the healthy alternative to stuffing the feelings down, ensures a healthy relationship to food. The healthy alternative can be described as allowing yourself to feel your feelings, acknowledging your feelings as important and taking appropriate action in line with healing those feelings and issues. We really do have two choices (a) to suppress our feelings and emotional issues or (b) experience and integrate them. Our goal as recovering compulsive eaters is to switch from (a) to (b).

Do not strike down every healthy suggestion that comes to mind when you ask yourself – Given the fact I feel this way what would I like to do now? Rather notice which ideas or suggestions appeal to you and try them out. Do not let irrational fears stop you. Instead simply notice your fears, analyse them as best you can and if they are irrational then as in the title of Susan Jeffers' famous self-help bible - Feel the Fear and Do It Anyway!
You also may have feelings of inadequacy, try to remember who planted those ideas originally in your head and move past them as best you can.
There also may be feelings of anger. Feeling like hitting your spouse is one to obviously <u>not</u> act on. Appropriate action in that case would be to really acknowledge the state of your relationship and take a brisk walk around the block even if you do not feel like walking, beat pillows or a mattress with your fists (even though it feels foolish) until the anger dissipates, or arrange to stay at a friend's house or hotel for a few days, even though you may not feel like taking that big of a step. Violence

must never be acted out, either towards yourself or another. There is always another way.

## (A) Suppressing feelings

Unresolved emotional issue and uncomfortable feelings.
Desire to suppress feelings / craving food when physically full.
Give in to craving, indulge in addiction, eat even though full.
Feeling is suppressed, physical discomfort of being too full.
Feelings of guilt and remorse.
Possibly induce vomiting or take laxatives.
Feelings and emotional issue remains suppressed, unresolved and still a problem, you still suffer from an eating disorder, more weight is gained.

## (B) Feeling, experiencing and integrating feelings

Unresolved emotional issue and uncomfortable feelings.
Desire to suppress feelings, craving to eat when physically full.
Acknowledge craving. Acknowledge physical fullness.
Ask: What feeling is this? Allow yourself to feel that feeling.
Ask: Given the fact I feel this way, what would I like to do now?
Listen to and follow the healthy ideas and guidance.
That healthy guidance leads to the resolving of your emotional issues. Thus you heal your eating disorder.
The power to be or not to be a food addict is within you.
The addicted relationship to food is replaced by a healthy, non-addicted one when we stop using food to suppress our feelings, and we begin to feel and integrate our feelings. Here are two

paths open to everyone — The path of integration (life-enhancing) and the path of suppression (self-defeating). Each path has its characteristics. Read on and decide which path you want to choose.

## Suppression v Integration

**Suppression is self-defeating behaviour and involves the following:**

<u>Taking unhealthy risks.</u> For a food addict it is repeatedly eating even though you are already physically full of food, causing excess weight, eating 'unhealthy' food which, over time especially, can make you unhealthy. For other addicts it is activities such as drug taking, staying with an abusive partner, drinking or smoking; even greed is an addiction, wanting more and more money, power, control over others — all detrimental.

<u>Self-hate</u> or self-loathing is a common feeling that food addicts have towards their bodies.

<u>Self-abuse</u>. It is a self-abusive activity to stuff more and more food into an already full stomach.

<u>Ill health</u> follows in the form of excess weight and various other related illnesses.

<u>Nausea</u> after a binge. This of course is unhealthy and uncomfortable.

<u>Blocked in life</u>. If we block our emotions, it follows that we are setting up energy blocks in our life that can manifest as financial,

career, health or relationship blocks. Life stays in the same old rut or gets worse instead of healthily moving forward.

<u>Relying on old negative patterns</u> of behaviour to deal with emotional issues. Eating when physically full is the familiar, old, dysfunctional method we may have learned from parents or picked up in childhood and adolescence as a way to cope.

<u>Emotional issues remain unresolved</u>. Emotional issues must come out of suppression and into the light of awareness to be faced up to and dealt with in healthy ways in order to be resolved. Eating when full prevents this natural healing and resolving to take place.

<u>Stuffing feelings down with food</u>. Eating when full stuffs our emotions and feelings down below our level of conscious awareness.

<u>Rejecting feelings</u>. Running away from and avoiding feelings Avoiding reality. Not relating to life as it is.

<u>Refusing to change what can be changed</u>. Refusing to do the emotional work to heal the past traumas and change what needs to be changed in one's own life, such as leave a marriage, get a job, file for a divorce or seek an education.

<u>Not in tune with your needs</u> and not meeting your needs appropriately (both emotional and physical).

<u>Suppressing your creativity</u>. We are all creative beings and following your likes, your interests and spending some time involved in what you love doing and feel is important to you, is a must to leading a life free from compulsive eating.

<u>Not aware of your inner self</u>, not in integrity. Your inner self is your feeling nature, your likes and dislikes, and integrity comes from honouring your inner self. Doing what another wants you to do when it is not what you want to be doing, is being out of integrity, and it is basically lying to yourself, not standing up for yourself and what is important to you. Allowing people to walk all over you or staying where someone is repeatedly mistreating you or tricking you, is a lack of integrity and will lead to binge eating or other addictions quite easily.

<u>Ignoring your innermost healthy desires</u> leading to feelings of unhappiness and dissatisfaction.

Food eaten when full is the object of addiction.

## Integration is life-enhancing behaviour and involves the following:

<u>Taking healthy risks</u> such as joining that art class you've wanted to join for years.

<u>Self-forgiveness</u> is acknowledging the times we have hurt others and made mistakes, it is a vow to cleanse out negative feelings that deplete us, and commit to changing our behaviour so we become kinder, wiser, stronger people with self-acceptance and self-respect.

<u>Uplifted, positive</u> state of mind.

<u>Stopping eating when full.</u> Good digestion. Not drinking alcohol or smoking. Not indulging in other addictions. Has healthy relationships and friendships. Overall good health.

<u>Using holistic ways</u> of dealing with emotional issues. Ways that do not involve the suppression of the issue.

<u>Emotional issues constantly get resolved</u>. Feelings are felt. Feelings are integrated. Moving forward in life.

<u>Finding and using</u> new healthy appropriate ways to deal with feelings, emotions and old traumas.

<u>Accepting feelings</u> and emotions rather than judging them. Accepting and dealing with reality as it is.

<u>Taking steps to change</u>, and actually changing what can be changed in terms of your own habits, patterns of behaviour and life situations.

<u>In tune with your own needs</u> (emotional, physical and spiritual). Meeting those needs in healthy appropriate ways.

<u>Expanding your creativity.</u> Join that evening class that you've wanted to join for years, (language, art or pottery for example). Following, becoming involved in your interests for that is expanding your creativity.

<u>Food becomes a pleasure</u> that simply provides nourishment for the body, as opposed to the object of an addiction.

Why should we stay on the more negative of those two paths when it looks so detrimental and unpleasant? Well, the negative, self-defeating path is probably the one you are more familiar with. It is the one you know, having been given an unhealthy psychological blueprint by a dysfunctional family as a child. In case you feel that is too harsh, don't worry, most families, to a greater or lesser extent are dysfunctional. An unpleasant truth, but a truth that explains the pandemic of obesity and addiction that is the reality of the planet today. It is not our fault nor our parents fault that what we once considered to be normal healthy behaviour was, in fact, dysfunctional. If your parents kept feeding you way past the stage of being physically full, they most likely did it in all innocence, genuinely wanting the best for you. Likewise, if they always offered you food instead of showing you real love and affection, they probably did it unconsciously and simply did not know of any other way to comfort you or show you love, echoes of their own upbringing.

Now we realise where our patterns originated, we let go of blame, simply understanding the facts. Blame is for victims. You choose not to be a victim the moment you take responsibility for your own health and healing. The point I wish to reinforce here is that it is our responsibility to learn how to break out of those inappropriate ways of feeding ourselves so that we are no longer food addicts. We can then begin to live a healthy fulfilling life where our children can develop and grow with the same freedom from addiction that we can enjoy as healed adults.

## We have a power point

That power point is the point when we are physically full. From being physically full we can choose the healthy, non-addicted, life-enhancing path which involves not eating again until actually physically hungry. Or, we can chose the path of addiction, self-defeating behaviour and eating even though we are already physically full.

We all have a part of ourselves that is like a child demanding food even though she is already physically full. This is what happens at the power point. You are already physically full but that inner child is screaming for cakes and stuffing in the food even though she is physically full. The remedy? How would you talk to your own child if she was demanding food when full? Would you allow her to keep on eating in a way that would make her bloated, sick and overweight? Would you ignore her compulsive behaviour? Of course not. You would ask her: What is wrong honey? Is something bothering you because you said you were already full up and there is no need to eat more if you are already full up. Did anything happen to upset you? You do not have to eat that way, let's see if we can make things better. What would you like to do? Go for a walk to the park? Tell me what is bothering you. I am here for you. If your tummy is already full then you don't really want that food; what do you really want and we'll see if we can get it. What do you really want? What would you like to do now? And let's do it!

Do the same for yourself. Ask yourself these self-same questions. You can ask yourself aloud in private or quietly in your thoughts, but ask you must. This suppressed compulsive child part of you has never been given any appropriate attention. This is an emotional gap. A lack of love and understanding, which caused you pain, fear and anger. Having no outlet for these feelings you suppressed them and are still suppressing them. They will stay suppressed until you fill in that emotional gap through appropriately relating to yourself and your inner child.

## We can fill in those emotional gaps

Now, in order to heal, you can listen with love and understanding to this previously neglected inner child. Calm your inner child and that compulsive part of you that is crying out to be healed. Actively encourage that healing through nurturing yourself and asking yourself appropriate questions. The appropriate questions that a caring, loving, emotionally present parent would ask their child if she was obviously behaving in a compulsive way. This child may be very unruly and compulsive but with loving attention and nurturing you can heal your inner child, so she becomes the healthy, happy child within.

Do not criticise, scold or threaten your inner child. That kind of treatment may have been partially to blame for her present compulsive behaviour and it certainly will not help you heal right now. Rather, lovingly open up a dialogue with your inner child. Ask some of those suggested questions and a few more besides. Reassure her. Tell her you love her and forgive her. Show her how to heal with this newfound knowledge you have. Encourage her to eat when she is physically hungry and stop when physically full. Allow her to play and explore her likes and dislikes. Let her try new things, because ultimately, she is you. Help her tune into her feelings and resolve those feelings. Boost her self-acceptance by telling her all the reasons she should love and accept herself right now, the way she is. Tell her she is wonderful, for that is the truth about her. Reassure her that she can heal and she is going to feel much better soon. Tell her, the pain does go away. Tell her, you love her and accept her as she is now. Let her know that you are there for her. Be her loving, wise parent, for in so doing you are becoming you own loving, wise parent. This is essential to healing your eating habit – the habit of eating when full.

Giving yourself the love and affection, the respect and acknowledgement that you did not get as a child, is what I call filling in the gaps. Filling in those inner, empty spaces left over from childhood. The gaps which are the results of lack. Lack of love. Lack of approval. Lack of reassurance. Lack of praise. Lack of harmony. Lack of respect. Lack of hugs and kisses from parents or caregivers. This lack, this emotional vacuum can be filled from within by you giving to your inner child. You giving to you. In truth, only when you are able to reassure, accept and approve of yourself, can you really begin to recognise and receive it from others.

Learning how to give to yourself unconditional love, reassurance, praise and approval, fills in your own personal emotional gaps. Learning how to deal with your emotional issues and feelings appropriately, fills in those gaps. Gaps which compulsive eaters try to fill in with food. Food cannot heal these emotional wounds. Meeting your own emotional needs appropriately, does, in a beautifully effective way!

Affirmation – Divine Love comes from an eternal and infinite source. Divine Love is the answer. Divine Love gives me unconditional love day and night. Divine Love heals me and empowers me to be the person I desire to be. Divine Love is within me. I am surrounded by Divine Love. I dwell in Divine Love and Divine Love dwells in me. I am healed, thank goodness I am healed!

As you give up compulsive eating, you are becoming more experienced at feeling your feelings. You are also becoming more aware of your thoughts and beliefs. You are able to distinguish between self-defeating thoughts and beliefs and life-enhancing thoughts and beliefs. Releasing what is self-defeating whilst embracing and adopting what is life-enhancing as your permanent positive belief system.

As far as feelings are concerned, you can discover and experiment with the thoughts and beliefs that can best help you deal with any uncomfortable feelings, and still not feel too overwhelmed by these new and sometimes strange emotions that you had previously kept firmly under wraps by eating when full.

You are becoming aware that you can even change an uncomfortable feeling, into a more positive one, just by thinking more positive thoughts. You are realising that by reassuring yourself and repeating a positive thought that you begin to believe it. You maybe even, have had the experience of repeating a positive statement, and seeing positive results in direct relation to that statement become a reality in your life. This points you towards the idea of how powerful your thoughts, beliefs and feelings really are, what an effect they have on your reality and the all-important realisation that your thoughts and beliefs are under your control. And how you deal with your feelings i.e. binge and suppress, or feel and integrate, is also under your control.

## Fulfilling your potential

Failing to fulfil your potential can contribute to you becoming addicted to food when full or other substances. In fact, I am convinced that addiction is a means of coping with a life that we are not yet completely satisfied with, and in which we are not yet fulfilling our own unique potential.

Often the addict has a sense of hopelessness about the possibility of changing her life into a life she can be happy with. Dealing with hopelessness and shame are often issues for healing addicts. Even guilt about wanting to enjoy a better way of life and feelings of not deserving that better lifestyle are also key issues that come up again and again for the healing addict. Indulging in addiction may be the only thing that comes close to being a pleasurable experience. Remember, if you are regularly eating when full and carry excess weight, you are a food addict. Food when full is your fix, the fix you crave; observing your own eating habits and cravings and you will notice this to be true.

Once you have learned how to deal with your feelings of guilt and shame (for example, through affirmation, positive thinking or breath work) and overcome any doubts about being worthy of a good life and good health – what next? Well, you start out on the life-long road of fulfilling your own potential. And the best way to make that start is, to ask yourself these questions: What would I like my life to be like? What job would I like to do? What kind of relationship do I want? And – How would I like to spend my time?

This is the time to think in unlimited ways. In the rubbish bin with the – Yes but's and the shoulds. Make lists of what you desire to do and be. Make lists of what you love to do in life. Write down your dreams. Visualise what your ideal life would be like. Remember, no limitations. As my friend's mother used to say - There is no tax on dreaming! That means, just enjoy visualising what you want without restriction, as if nothing can stop you, and there are no obstacles. Don't get depressed if your visualisation is vastly different to your present reality. It's bound to be! They are not to be compared. Understand, that visualising your desired reality daily, does indeed change you on an inner level, bringing you into mental and emotional harmony with that precious goal. As a result you become open and receptive to new ideas and opportunities concerning your goal that may never have occurred otherwise.

Feelings help propel thoughts and beliefs into reality! So, empower yourself! If you desire to be slim start to feel slim. If you desire to be a career woman imagine what it would feel like to be a career woman. Play with your imagination. Allow yourself to be a modern day magician. Wave your magic wand

and mentally declare to yourself – Now, now I am slim. And feel what it is like to be slim. Experience slimness. Embrace the good feelings. If you desire a larger income – feel what it is like to have a larger income, knowing that you can buy whatever you want, live wherever you want, and be debt free. Let all the feelings be positive and if any fearful or unpleasant feelings slip in, reassure yourself that you can deal with those fears too.

On a practical level, do what you can to help yourself feel you are approaching your goal. You can take courage and take action. Take those small steps toward the life you really desire. This may mean enrolling in a night class, or devoting a half hour or more a day to something you really love such as writing, meditating, painting or baking.

When we are busy fulfilling our potential – doing what we love, actively working towards having the life we want, being around people we love and meeting the challenges of our day to day lives - we feel useful, fulfilled, challenged, satisfied and empowered. It is challenging and involves daring to be the unique you, the real you, if you like, instead of the you waiting to be slim enough or rich enough to live! It is, in no uncertain terms, rewarding – the path of meeting your own emotional needs and fulfilling your own unique potential. This contributes greatly to humanity being full of healthy individuals as opposed to addicted individuals.

So by now you know that fulfilling your potential includes meeting your emotional needs appropriately. Acknowledging your own needs and meeting them appropriately leads to a happy life. The need to be loved is satisfied by good friends and being in a healthy, loving, intimate relationship or marriage, where both partners are healthy, non-addicted, self-accepting individuals who simply reflect each other's own sense of self-worth and integrity. They have a high regard for one another and are self-aware enough to be able to grow and heal any wounds that may surface during the relationship. If the relationship has run its course each one is financially and emotionally able to leave.

Another important human need is the need for shelter, warmth and comfort. The need to be comfortably housed is met by taking time and care when selecting a house or flat in which to live. Also allowing your gut instinct to tell you whether a place is right for you or not.

The need to have a feeling of belonging or a sense of community can come from work, hobbies or participation in local events or clubs.

The need for companionship, feeling supported and loved comes from having and developing healthy, nurturing friendships with like-minded souls. Take away any of these and you have a gap, an emotional gap and an unfulfilled need.

The need is not wrong nor there to be suppressed. The need is healthy. The fact that the need is not being met is the only unhealthy thing going on. So, if you find some emotional gaps, don't despair, the tools given throughout this book will help you fill in those gaps.

## Reclaiming our power around food

When food is your only means of coping with emotional issues, it is you that is giving food that power. Some people find it hard to believe that they actually do have a choice in this, simply because of their strong feelings of having no choice, or being out of control and powerless around food. This all changes in the course of recovery.

I have mentioned this before but it bears repeating as it is paramount that you fully grasp this fact – The compulsive behaviour is optional. Your power point is where you choose either the obsessive, compulsive, self-defeating behaviour or the life-enhancing, healthy, experiencing your feelings, behaviour. Your specific point of power around food is when you are physically full yet still crave to eat more. Your choice being: to eat even though you are physically full (self-defeating) or wait until physically hungry before eating (life-enhancing) and asking yourself our habit busting questions – What feeling is this? And given the fact I feel this way, what would I like to do now? Remembering all this helps you reclaim your power for accurate knowledge is power.

## Why we feel powerless around food

What makes us feel powerless around food is our addiction to it. Recognising your sense of powerlessness around food is one of the first steps in healing, in that once you realise this, you are no longer in denial of the problem. In fact, you are recognising that there is a problem of power and control laced with underlying emotional issues and cravings.

**What keeps us addicted is:**
1.   The lack of accurate knowledge about the true dynamics of our problem.
2.   Treating the symptom (the excess weight) rather than treating the cause (the unresolved emotional issues).
3.   Not knowing what healthy alternative way could best help us feel and integrate our feelings.
4.   Knowing the healthy alternative ways of dealing with feelings but being unable to incorporate those healthy alternative ways into our day to day life because of resistance.

Remember, compulsive eating or our addiction to food, is only one way to deal with a life with which we are not yet completely satisfied. The process of finding, experimenting with and incorporating into our day to day lives the healthy alternatives to stuffing down our feelings is the process of reclaiming our power over the object of our addiction – food when full.

Affirmation – There is nothing for me to fear. I am regaining my power over food. I now stop eating when full.

If you do eat when full forgive yourself, for this is a step by step journey where setbacks, road blocks and wrong turns are part of the adventure. Simply look at and resolve the feelings and emotional issues that drove you to eat when full that time.

Let us, for a moment look at a drug addict's life. Her whole existence is taken up with the satisfying of her compulsion to suppress the unpleasant feelings which she does not know how else to deal with. Her day is spent in the pursuit of the one thing that she knows will enable her to feel 'normal' and get rid of the feelings which she finds unbearable to experience. These unbearable feelings are, in my opinion, the dreaded withdrawal symptoms or cold turkey, which in truth are unresolved issues and unhealed traumas of the addict's past. I regard what is called 'withdrawal symptoms' to be more of an unrecognised and unresolved intensely painful issue or series of issues, events and situations with feelings to match. So what is called a withdrawal symptom is actually more of a root cause that surfaces once there is no drug-taking to suppress it.

Thankfully now, with greater knowledge of what in fact, addiction is, we know that recovery from addiction through the healing of the root cause makes withdrawal less painful. It is done holistically and relatively comfortably especially through energy healing, rebirthing breathwork and AA meetings.

So how do food addicts compare to drug addicts? I raise this question of comparison to emphasise how detrimental any addiction is, and to de-stigmatise drug addiction as the real 'baddie' in society. The root cause of addiction is the real culprit here and the lack of holistic healing methods and preventative methods that is where the finger of blame can be accurately pointed if any finger pointing is to be done. But ultimately self-responsibility is the only answer. Addiction itself an innocent by product, if you like, of the suppressed trauma. What causes traumas, who causes traumas, how to prevent traumas and how to heal traumas are the intelligent questions whose answers will provide a world free from addiction. That would be a completely different world I assure you.

Imagine, on your bus or train ride to work you see an advertisement display with your favourite positive quote or advertising the local community, holistic centre, free therapies available 24/7. Imagine advertising space devoted to helping, encouraging and highlighting health and healing as not only possible, but probable for everyone who has issues in their lives that they feel unable to adequately handle. What is also needed today is widespread information on how to deal with dysfunctional family behaviour. Most soaps, dramas and films show dysfunctional, even dangerous human relationships. A healthy soap would not be boring, but informative and a role model for health and vitality. And remember addiction to food when full or any other addiction is a means of coping with those dysfunctional relationships depicted as the norm. Knowledge combined with practice is our greatest healer.

The truth is, that drug addiction is no better or worse than any of the other addictions, that we all have available to us, as a means of dealing with our unresolved emotional issues. In fact, in some cases and some environments addiction is actively encouraged. This phenomenon occurs where most, or all, of the people in that environment happen to be addicted to one thing or another. Addiction therefore being the norm. In these cases the person who is no longer a drug addict, will stick out like the proverbial sore thumb, in her sobriety, when hanging out with stoned friends. An ex-workaholic going home at 5pm when the rest of the office is still slaving away. The ex-smoker refusing a fag. The ex-drinker, drinking orange juice in the pub. Needless to say we usually outgrow these environments as soon as we learn how to happily refuse the object of our addiction. It has simply run its course in our life.

Often we hear of one addiction being played off against another, stating with vigour that drug addiction should be condemned, and eradicated simply by withdrawing the object of addiction. This is unrealistic and ineffective. Addiction cannot be healed that way, because the underlying issues that drove her to the drugs remain unresolved. If these underlying emotional issues remain unresolved, we still have a problem. The one and only permanent cure for addiction involves the resolving of emotional issues and the experiencing of previously suppressed feelings. This willingness to feel one's own painful feelings, this willingness to experience the withdrawal symptoms (such as in a breathwork session) is what causes the integration or healing of these difficult feelings. Once we have integrated something we are no longer suppressing it, we no longer crave the activity (such as eating when full, drug taking or drinking alcohol).

Once we have integrated something, we no longer, consciously or subconsciously need to suppress it, we no longer crave to suppress it, hence we no longer crave that which enabled us to suppress it. Therefore we no longer need or crave drugs, food when full, cigarettes or alcohol. The root cause has been healed. So I will repeat - Forced deprivation of the object of addiction does little to help. It only causes the addict to experience the withdrawal symptoms or painful unresolved emotional issues without a healthy alternative way of dealing with them. The power to heal addiction lies, to a great extent, in the incorporation of that healthy alternative into daily life. When an addict chooses to cease her indulgence in drugs and with the aid of a good breathwork coach, therapist or group such as NA, the drug addict can heal permanently those original traumas and emotional issues, the root causes, and thus, in so doing, heals the addiction – the symptom of those root causes.

Unresolved issues, suppressed feelings caused by past dysfunctional or traumatic happenings, carry addiction as their ugly symptom. Thank goodness, through individuals healing, society is healed of addiction and its related problems.

## Surrounded by addiction?

In the world around us, food addiction and cigarette smoking may not even be noticed, understood or addressed as important. An alcoholic may be viewed with pity, but excessive drinking seen as somewhat acceptable. Being a shopaholic may be dismissed, and workaholism may be seen as a normal activity encouraged by some companies. What is important, is to be aware of what dynamic is operating in your environment and how it is effecting you. If you are a recovering addict you may find yourself becoming more aware of the addicted tendencies of those around you. It can be disconcerting at first. You may have the feeling of going against the grain. What is important to remember here is just to allow yourself to feel your feelings and act on them in appropriate ways. You may move house, emigrate or stay in the same place, whilst following your feelings and intuitive guidance. That does not matter. As you continue healing, growing, following your joy, doing what you love as much as you can, overcoming fear and self-doubt, being ever-vigilant for, and refusing to give in to, your own compulsive urges, you will sooner or later be led to a feeling of oneness, and contentment with your surroundings. We welcome the day when we look around, and see nothing but strong, healthy, loving individuals who are, in truth, our mirrors, reminding us of how much healing we have, in fact, done.

## About people around us suppressing their feelings

You know an addict is someone who suppresses what she cannot deal with in any other way. If you are a healthy person or a recovering addict (and remember that also means recovering from your habit of eating food when full) you may find yourself feeling suddenly angry or sad when you are with other people. The way you will know if someone around you is suppressing their feelings, is to physically move away from that person and notice if the feelings of anger or sadness subside. By being close to them you were literally picking up on, and maybe even absorbing the very emotions they suppress. These invisible dynamics are not well known in the world but they do exist.

Again, I will remind you that addiction is not the main source of our problem here. Addiction is a problem in itself, but it is also the symptom of a deeper problem. That deeper problem is all those suppressed feelings and emotional issues.

Another real concern is – Do the addicts around us have the desire to heal? If they do not, it can be emotionally draining for the recovering addict to be around such people. Distancing yourself from such people is fine.

However, if addicts do genuinely want to heal, then, the question is – Are the resources, knowledge and support systems sufficient to enable them to heal with the utmost ease? Do healing addicts have all the encouragement and support they need in order to see them through to complete recovery? Does society provide this support? You might be the one to give them a kind word or piece of important information as to how to heal. A book suggested can be the start of their own healing journey. But do not force information on people. Your intuition will guide you as to who is ready to heal and who is not, who is willing to listen and who simply does not want to know about addiction healing modalities.

And I do believe the resources are there. The one willing to heal may have to look hard to find them, it may not be easy, but the steady growth of these resources is happening, and surely can be a predominant part of every community, all over the world. The accessibility of self-help books, which can be either bought or borrowed from the local library, is increasing all the time. Being in therapy is no longer something of a stigma but rather seen as the healthy, practical way of enabling one to cope with the pressure of modern living. The success of AA, Al-Anon and NA speaks for itself.

Everyone is appreciating that a better way of life and good health is what they want and deserve. To a certain extent, a re-defining and a de-tabooing of addiction is necessary in order to allow healing to be more realistic and possible without any shame of saying – 'I'm a recovering / recovered addict.' This firstly occurs within each individual, as one by one we make the simple realisation that addiction is addiction, it is about suppressing feelings, and we can choose to feel, heal and integrate those feelings instead of suppressing them. In other words the healing of your own addiction, whatever it may be, is certainly possible and most importantly, starts with you!

## If the real problem is not drug addiction then what is?

Again, any addiction is both a problem within itself and it is also the symptom of a deeper problem. That deeper problem is not only the unresolved emotional issue but also our inability to deal with that issue in an appropriate, healthy way. Our real problem is the unhealed events and treatment, which caused us very real emotional suffering.

The way we were treated at birth and during childhood had, of course, tremendous impact in forming our first conclusions about life – life-long conclusions that became a blueprint for future events and a filter through which we view the world. Thankfully, through rebirthing and other techniques we can now access and change deep seated self-defeating, conclusions and filters to more life-affirming ones. That goes a long way to produce a healthier, happier, addiction-free life.

Rebirthing breathwork, positive thinking, energy healing and the like all are important parts of healing addiction for they help us feel and resolve deeply uncomfortable feelings caused by past traumas.

The painful feelings from past traumas, once resolved, empower us. So that, what was once trauma becomes an event from which we have graduated, if you like, gleaned a blessing in that it did not kill us or cause us to be addicts. A painful experience overcome, and injustice conquered, you emerge victorious and that is a mini miracle wouldn't you say?!

## Food addicts compared to drug addicts

Do you spend most of your day thinking about food, diets or your weight? We all know how obsessive food addiction can be and how much time is spent thinking about food and losing weight. So, like our fellow suppresser, the drug addict, our negative patterns of behaviour can cause our lives to be filled with the object of our addiction; thinking about the food, the diet, the ideal weight and getting special food for the diet, following the diet (staying sober) until we snap and dive into the food when full (drugs) to suppress our feelings that flow forth when there is no food when full or drugs to keep them firmly under wraps. A full life? Filled with activity, but hardly rewarding.

## Reasons for staying on that unhealthy path

Comfortable in its familiarity, others we know, are all doing the same. We share the activity like a form of bonding but it has no meaning, no depth, just shallow, instant, inappropriate ease from our unresolved issues, feelings, withdrawal symptoms and pain. We are all in the same club – The Big Girls Club – we have camaraderie don't we? Maybe unconsciously we have concluded that we don't have to deal with the unwanted attention or demands made on the beautiful, slim, stereotypical woman. We will never be her, she is to be despised as one who obviously has it all, yet paradoxically seems to have been hammered into a tiny role of female, silent, servitude to 'attractiveness'. We, on the other hand, in our size, rebel against the shallow stereotype of womanhood, we share the hidden pain of rejection and insecurity about our role in life, motherhood and men. Are we really second class citizens because of our gender? Were we denied real love and approval from our mothers because they had unresolved issues of not being respected and not being cared for? Because underneath it all, we women were supposed to be the carers of the world, not living breathing, thinking, dreamers of our own life. Is *being big* an unconscious attempt to *be big* in the daunting world? Is carrying excess weight a great big 'F\*\*k You' to everything and everyone that caused us pain? These may be deeper issues that are hidden from our conscious awareness as compulsive eaters, but as with any addict the addiction sets the addict apart from the norm, gives her some room to be different and experiment with a new paradigm for living. Who would you be if you stepped out of any role that you find distasteful? Who would you be if you got all the support, money and freedom you needed? Who would you be if you got your needs met?

Many people consider food addiction different from alcohol abuse or drug addiction, simply because food (the object of our addiction) is something from which we cannot abstain. However, what we are learning to abstain from is not food but eating food when physically full.

It varies from individual to individual, but in general, when the craving strikes, a compulsive eater can abstain from eating when physically full, with about as much ease as a recovering alcoholic or drug addict can abstain from indulging in the object of her addiction. Craving is craving, and it can have a weak, or powerful hold on you no matter what the craving is for. The key however, for breaking the craving is the same – pinpoint and heal the underlying, unresolved emotional pain.

## Eating whatever you want when physically hungry

Eat whatever you want when physically hungry. There are no good foods and no bad foods. If you fancy a doughnut or a slice of cream cake, it is fine to eat it once you are physically hungry. This way, you are giving you back the control.

Most of you, who have food and weight problems, feel like you are out of control around food. This is perfectly logical considering food is the object of your addiction. It may feel like food has the power to make you feel good. Having a good day or a bad day, for a compulsive eater, is often determined by how much food and the type of food eaten. For some of you a good day could mean eating hardly anything. A bad day could be a day when you broke the diet, had a binge, or ate 3 calories more than a designated amount – making you feel guilty, disappointed, helpless and angry at yourself, feeling you have failed. These feelings, in and of themselves, sometimes triggering yet another binge - and the cycle continues. But you must not blame yourself, it is what it is, a cycle that has deeper dynamics at play. Dynamics that through this book we are exploring and in understanding them, you can gain increased freedom and ability to say no to food when full and break that cycle of overeating.

Most of you agree that food has magical qualities and symbolic meanings. A piece of chocolate is a treat. Even in advertisements, cream cakes have been described as naughty but nice. The idea of food, especially sweet foods as a treat has been around for a long time and it is true to a certain extent. Food is pleasurable. Eating whatever you fancy when physically hungry, is not only an everyday treat, but a source of culinary satisfaction. However, it is necessary that we learn to treat ourselves in other more appropriate ways when physically full, thus making sure that food isn't our only treat.

## Mixed messages or what!

Along with a family history of mixed messages, like: 'Eat up but be slim,' the media images only add to our confusion. After all, when did you last see a larger than size 10 woman in a fashion magazine, on the catwalk or drinking a diet soda on a TV ad?

The diet ads especially are selling you the same thing as this book is selling you – a slim figure. Only I am giving you a lot more knowledge about how you gained the weight in the first place and the true nature of your eating / weight problem. I also feel that the contents of this book are a far more empowering than the short, sharp glamor burst of the TV ad, diet product.

Advertisements tend to be glamorous and appealing. They are supposed to be, and therefore can be taken with a pinch of salt. The advertisement will hit you in all the right places psychologically in order to sell its product. The truth is, diet products and diets are ineffective mainly because they focus on the surface symptom – the excess weight - rather than the real problem, the unresolved emotional issues. They imply if the outer appearance is okay then you'll be okay. Fix the outer and the inner happiness is found, but the truth is - Fix the inner, heal your inner, emotional world and the outer reflection falls into place.

My opinion, on diet foods, is the same as with all food – if you are genuinely, physically hungry and you fancy eating it, then eat it, and stop when you are physically full. I personally love the taste and texture of certain diet crackers and add them to my shopping list.

I also encourage you to keep your favourite foods in the kitchen! Eating what you want, when you want, once you are physically hungry is made easier by having an ample larder. Yes, that means stock up on that deadly chocolate ice cream, your favourite cheese, crackers, the crisps, cream cakes, frozen chips or whatever it is that you have been busily denying yourself over the past few years or more.

A lot of women fear doing this, simply because they feel that they would not be able to resist eating all this food, and as a result, gain even more weight. A natural and understandable fear. However, what we are doing, when we fill our kitchen cabinets and fridges with our favourite foods, is facing that fear. We are learning to trust ourselves around food. We are testing our ability to eat when hungry and stop when full by having all the tempting food around. We are affirming that we deserve to have the food we love in the house, available to us when we are hungry. We are displaying a trust in ourselves to nourish our bodies appropriately. For the truth of the matter is, that if we do manage to eat only when physically hungry and stop when physically full, even though all that tempting food is in the house, then we really have healed our addiction to food.

Let's also remind ourselves that controlling our food intake, through forced denial of our favourite foods, does not help us to heal our addiction to food. Those kind of thoughts helped start it! You bring choice into the equation to free things up and help release you from your obsession. It is quite hard to be obsessed with something when you are trusting yourself around the object of your obsession, pondering your choices as to whether it is wise to indulge in it and have learned about the true nature of your obsession.

## Follow the threads to your slim-self

I would like you to imagine that you are already your slim-self, and I would like you to ask yourself the following questions:
Remember, answer these questions as if you are already your desired weight.
Are you your perfect weight?
Do you accept your size and shape completely?
Can you wear the clothes you want to wear?
Do you enjoy life?
Do you have a partner?
Do you like your body?
What job do you do?
How do you spend your time?
Is there anything negative in your life?
Now comes the tricky bit! Look at your answers and either change your perception so that they could be true for you now or ask yourself - What could I do to make that answer true for me now? In effect you are asking yourself what would making them true, involve regardless of what size I am? Remember getting slim alone will not necessarily bring these things to you.
Here are some examples:
Do I accept my size and shape completely?
My slim-self says - Yes

Question - What could I do to make that 'yes' true for me now? Answer – I would have to do a lot of self-acceptance affirmations. I could cease criticising myself and praise myself a little instead.

Do I enjoy life?
My slim-self says – Yes
Question – What could I do to make that 'yes' true for me now?
Answer - I could make a list of and start to do more of the activities I love.

Are you your perfect weight?
My slim-self says – Yes
Question – How can I change my perception of my weight to make this true for mem now?
Answer – I may think that at the smaller size I have the right to say – I am my perfect weight now – however, at the larger size I am now, can I still say it? Of course I can! My weight is the perfect expression of all those times I stuffed my feelings down with food when full. It is the perfect, albeit unwanted, results of the difficult events in my past and my way of coping with them. When I was angry at my mother and ate half that fruit pie, felt positively stuffed and then some! That is there. Perfectly accurately recorded in my fat cells. Not very perfect you might say. However, this eating food when I am not even physically hungry is the perfect way for me to deal with my feelings when I do not know how else to deal with them. Inappropriate – Yes.

Is there a slim-friendly way that I may adopt in the future second, minute or hour? Yes! (in this book). But for now, or in the past, eating when full and excess weight was the perfect expression of who I was with the knowledge I had! – Yes! With this change of perception – Yes, I am my perfect size and shape for me now! It is my past way of eating that got me like this, and I can change – Yes!

As with self-acceptance, if you cannot see the perfection in your present, larger size and shape, you could also be faced with the reality of being blind to the perfection of your slimmer size and shape too.

I have learned that the ability to see perfection is not inexorably linked with a certain dress size; we all know there are many slim women who still complain about their slim bodies.

Understand that changing your perception is the purpose of this lesson. The more your thinking is the same whether you are fat or slim, the more you are following those threads of similarity from the reality of being fat to the reality of being slim.

## Map your progress from larger size not recovered to smaller size completely recovered.

Characteristics of larger size not recovered:

1. Does not accept her size and shape.
2. Thinks life would be different or better if only she was slimmer.
3. Does not necessarily know when she is physically hungry. Sometimes does not eat when physically hungry. Often is in a

state of over-fullness. Does not know when physically full, or does recognise physical fullness but is totally unable to stop eating at that point.

4. Is unable to distinguish between physical and emotional hunger. Eats food when emotionally hungry. Eats when full. Does not know how to nourish herself on an emotional level. Often in abusive or dysfunctional relationships. Uses food to meet her emotional needs. Uses food when full to suppress her emotions.

5. Often eats foods she does not particularly want even though she is physically full. She eats regardless of whether she is physically full or not, simply because it is mealtime or because the food is just there.

6. She is waiting until she is slim before living the life she really wants to live. She is waiting until she is slim before wearing the clothes she really wants to wear. She is waiting until she is slim before working towards having the career or relationship she really wants to have.

7. Blames others for her problems. Blames circumstances for her life's problems. Avoids her feelings rather than feeling her feelings and taking responsibility for her life and it's challenges.

8. Feels out of control around food. Is afraid of food, in a love / hate relationship with food. Has an addicted relationship to food i.e. uses food to distance herself from her unresolved emotional issues.

9. Her body size is the result of her eating in order to suppress her feelings and emotional issues. It's size is a result of her addiction to food when full. The prospect of gaining or losing weight is fraught with emotion. Has conscious fears of becoming fatter and subconscious fears around becoming slim.

## Characteristics of larger size in the process of recovery:

1. She is learning how to accept her size and shape completely. Her self-acceptance is growing steadily. She is also learning how to accept her personality completely. She begins to acknowledge and appreciate herself, her body size, her own qualities as a human being as well as her own needs and desires spiritual, mental, emotional and physically.
2. She acknowledges the parts of herself she wants to change, like her size, aspects of her personality, areas of her life and she learns new tools which enable her to change that which she wants to change about herself and her life.
3. Becoming more aware of when physically hungry and almost always eats when physically hungry. Becoming more aware of when physically full and is almost always able to stop eating when physically full.
4. She is learning the difference between physical and emotional hunger. She is learning how to nourish herself emotionally.
5. She is learning how to eat exactly what she wants when she is physically hungry and often does so. Sometimes overeats or returns to old dysfunctional eating patterns but does not beat

herself up about it. She is learning to forgive herself rather than feel guilty. She notices how it feels physically to overeat and acknowledges that she is at the learning stage of recovery, learns from her experience and moves on.

6. Starts to ask herself what she really wants from life, relationships, career etc. She also asks herself what she wants to wear. She starts to live the life she wants to live now. She is developing the relationships, hobbies and career she wants.

7. She starts to accept more responsibility for her life, ceases to blame or finger point, instead she sees what she can do to achieve her goals.

8. She is beginning to feel more in control around food; food is losing its magic. She is beginning to enjoy food more as one of life's simple wholesome pleasures.

9. Her body is in the process of finding its own natural weight. The prospect of losing weight is no longer a major issue, rather an assured result. Gaining weight may still be fearful and she is in the process of resolving her conscious fears of weight gain and subconscious fears around weight loss.

10. She is trusting her body's needs much more now. Aware of those subtle hunger and fullness sensations more and more. Aware of her intuition more and more. Experimenting with how to respond to those needs appropriately. Experiencing satisfaction when discovering what works for her.

## Characteristics of larger size completely recovered:

1. Accepts her size and shape completely. Accepts all aspects of her personality completely.
2. Acknowledges the aspects of her life, herself and her personality that she wants to change and is in the process of changing them.
3. Knows when physically hungry and eats. Knows when physically full and stops eating.
4. Knows when emotionally hungry and nourishes herself emotionally.
5. Eats exactly what she wants when she wants as long as physically hungry.
6. Lives the life she wants to live now. Wears the clothes she wants to wear now. Has the career or works towards having the career she wants now. Has the relationship, or is working towards having the relationship she wants.
7. Accepts responsibility for herself and her life.
8. Feels perfectly happy and in control around food, has a healthy and natural, non-addicted relationship to food.
9. Her body is in the process of losing excess weight. Her body is finding and maintaining its own natural weight. The prospect of gaining or losing weight is not frightening but simply a necessary part of the body finding and maintaining its own natural weight in response to her changing eating habits.
10. She trusts her body's needs and responds to them appropriately (whether those needs are emotional, spiritual,

mental or physical she responds to those needs with respect, love and joy).

Note: The characteristics of larger size completely recovered is very similar to smaller size completely recovered. While still at the larger size we have completely adopted the characteristics of the completely healed compulsive eater. So in these lists of characteristics we are seeing the morphing of a compulsive eater into an person free from compulsive eating. Overlapping occurs and as with any recovered addict even when healed we must always be aware of the old habits sneaking back, so we can catch them, and address them and their deeper issues appropriately.

**Characteristics of smaller size completely recovered**

1. Accepts her size and shape completely. Accepts her personality completely.
2. Acknowledges the aspects of herself and her life which she wants to change and is in the process of changing them.
3. Knows when physically hungry and eats. Knows when physically full and stops eating.
4. Knows when emotionally hungry and nourishes herself emotionally.
5. Eats exactly what she wants when she wants as long as she is physically hungry.
6. Lives the life she wants to live now. Wears the clothes she wants to wear now. Has the career or works towards having the career she wants now. Has the relationship or works towards having the relationship she wants to have now.

7.     Accepts responsibility for her life and herself. Accepts the things she can't change, and changes the things she can change.
8.     Feels perfectly happy and in control around food. Enjoys food, has a healthy non-addicted relationship to food. Food is a pleasure and she has no fear around food.
9.     Her body has found and maintained its own natural weight. The prospect of gaining or losing weight is not frightening or a concern any more as she has developed a healthy trust in her bodily sensations of hunger and fullness.
10.    She trusts her body's needs and responds to them appropriately (whether those needs are emotional, mental, spiritual or physical she responds to them with respect love and joy).

## What are you afraid of?

Another important factor in losing weight permanently and healing your eating habit is to discover any subconscious fears around being slim. You can do this very easily with the help of the following visualisation. Before doing any visualisation it is a good idea to spend time quietening the mind and relaxing the body. Try this gentle relaxation technique before you visualise.

Make the setting as comfortable as beautiful as possible. Have your favourite objects near you such as a pretty ornament, some crystals, a vase of flowers or a lit candle. Have some spare cushions and a warm blanket for extra comfort. If you like, burn some incense and play some soft instrumental music. These things are not essential by any means, and you can do a perfectly good visualisation without them. Setting the scene and creating the atmosphere is completely up to you and can be a real treat when you desire to pamper yourself.

So now, whether you have set the scene or not, sit or lie down in a comfortable position and make sure you will not be disturbed for at least twenty minutes. And... let your toes and feet relax... relax your ankles... relax your legs... your calf muscles... allow your knees to relax... and your upper legs... your hips and thighs... allow your pelvis and buttocks to relax... relax your lower back and stomach... feel the tension flowing away from your body as you relax... allow your middle back relax... your ribcage and chest muscles relax... your upper back and shoulders relax... Feel the tension being released from your shoulders maybe move them gently a few times and hear them click out the stress and tension... Relax your neck and facial muscles, your jaw and scalp... completely relax... now do a quick scan of your body and notice if there is anywhere you are holding remaining tension and let it go. There is no right way or wrong way to do this, so do not worry, if you think of a muscle and gently mentally say to it 'relax' it will, to a greater or lesser extent it will relax and that is good enough.

Now visualise yourself in the following situation. You are at a dinner party with your closest friends and family... In a large and very beautiful house... in the centre of the dining room there is a large dining table with gold candlesticks with twinkling candles, crystal vases with the most beautiful flowers. The whole room is luxurious and richly decorated… How do you feel in this room, in such grand surroundings?

You and your friends sit down to eat… take your place at the head of the table… now check in with your stomach as it is now in reality… How hungry are you? Order food according to that hunger and what you fancy eating now, in reality… You can eat whatever you want… the menu is unlimited and the chefs are the best… Do not worry if you are not very hungry, this is a visualisation you can do daily or weekly to discover various degrees of hunger and fullness. If you are ravenous now have a feast, if you are not very hungry then eat according to that sensation of hunger and being just a bit peckish maybe all you want to have is crackers and cheese with a coffee. If you fancy something sweet have desert, the one of your choice. No one is going to scold you here, everyone is ordering what they want and you can too.

Notice how difficult or easy it is for you to make your food choices based on what your stomach is telling you. Notice the 'shoulds' that creep in or the judgements you feel you may get from others. What if I am full and just have a glass of water? What if I am starving and eat lots? Notice the thoughts and feelings around you having what you want in front of your friends and family in this lavish, abundant setting.

Now your food is ready, it magically appears in front of you… notice how it looks… as you eat notice how you feel towards your family and friends… Now I would like you to imagine you are getting fatter and fatter, at the same table with the same food, family and friends. Notice any differences, are you shy and vulnerable, or the life and soul of the dinner party, are you more talkative? Notice the clothes you are wearing now that you are larger than you have ever been before. Go beyond any negative feelings and see if you can find something positive in being this large lady at the dinner party. Does it give you some kind of strength or protection? There is a previously hidden positive aspect in being this large woman at the dinner party, what is it? It may take a few visualisations to find so do not worry too much. Now I would like you to imagine that you are losing all that excess weight, you are eating the same food with the same people at the same dinner. Notice any differences now that you are slim. Different reactions from your family and friends, different clothes you are wearing now you are slim? See if you can go beyond the happiness you feel at being your ideal weight, and see if you can find some previously hidden, negative aspect of being the slim, attractive woman at the dinner party. This is important for it is a hidden fear of being slim that in real life prevents you from losing excess weight for good, so really stay with it until you find what is a little scary in being slim. Allow the scene to fade and remember where you are, sitting in your room, maybe with your favourite items around, sitting in your chair or lying down, feel your head on the pillow and breathe deeply a few times, open your eyes and move slowly starting with your fingers and your toes, as you bring yourself out of the visualisation. Write down your insights. Good, well done. You have dipped into the waters and knowledge of your own subconscious to discover what will help you lose excess weight for good, namely the positive in being larger and the negative in being slim.

1. I can be slim and (positive aspect of being larger)
2. I promise to take my (positive aspect of being larger) with me when I get slim.
3. I am becoming more and more (positive aspect of being larger) every day.

## 'I am…' affirmations

Any affirmation containing the words 'I am' is particularly powerful. It is an ancient success secret, that the words 'I am' when spoken aloud, or written repeatedly, actively connects us with, and generates within us a powerful spiritual force for good. Even Moses demanding of Pharoah – Let my people go! (Exodus 5:1, 7:16) stated that 'I am' had sent him (Exodus 3:14). Experiment with it for yourself by affirming the following:

I am (positive aspect of being slim).
I am (positive aspect of being large).
I am becoming more and more… (positive aspects) …every day.

Use these affirmations 15 minutes daily. Think them, say them aloud in private or silently to yourself, write them out in a beautiful note book that you keep privately just for affirmations. Keep reminding yourself of their positive message throughout your day, and remind yourself, if their negative opposites arise (which may have been a previous form of thinking) that those old, negative, self-defeating thoughts are simply not true, until you find enough reasons for the positive truth to reign supreme in your mind and in your life.

For example: If you felt wonderfully confident when you visualised yourself slim, then confidence is your positive aspect of being slim and the appropriate I am affirmation would be - I am confident. If safety and security was the positive aspect that came up for you when you visualised yourself larger, then the appropriate affirmation would be - I am safe and secure.

Develop the positive attributes of yourself highlighted in the visualisation, through the repeated use of the 'I am' affirmations. Think 'I am confident' on the train to work, waiting for the bus, doing the dishes or brushing your teeth. Sounds ridiculous? No, telling yourself how lacking in confidence, how unattractive you are and other such cruel, negative thoughts, that's ridiculous! You will only make yourself miserable by thinking negatively rather than looking for and developing the positive, like a seed to a flower it takes time but results do come as you persist. So, think positive, think prosperous, think healthy, wealthy and wise. Give yourself your own vote of confidence. Remember, whatever you think being slim will give you, it is nothing that you cannot start developing within yourself today. So, start affirming that you already have that cherished quality. It is the repeated affirmation feeding your conscious and subconscious mind that waters the seed of that particular attribute to maturity. In other words, through repeating an affirmation of, let us say, confidence, daily, you allow the idea of confidence to sink into your subconscious mind, becoming something you believe possible for you (becoming part of your belief system) something you believe to a greater or lesser extent and thus becomes a reality in your life.

Our mind is like a computer. We feed in the command and it produces the appropriate information. We ask it a question and it comes up with an answer from its conscious, subconscious and even super-conscious data banks. If, in your data banks you have the piece of information saying - I am not confident – and you ask yourself a question such as - I wonder will I get that job I applied for? – your mind with its belief of no self-confidence may come up with doubts such as I am probably not the person they are looking for. There are probably going to give it to a younger, smarter, person. However, you could re-program your computer-like mind with – I am confident the job right for me now comes to me. And when you ponder – Will I get that job I applied for? – maybe your future could look brighter with the answer going something like – I am confident that I can succeed in life. I am confident that I can get this job and if I don't then I know it was simply not the right position for me and an even better one is on its way to me now.

Basically, whatever you believe, is what you will see before you in your life. Therefore, by becoming aware of what thoughts and belief systems are in your mind you can change the negative self-defeating beliefs to more positive, life-enhancing ones.

'Why should I do this?' You may ask. Well, negative thoughts and negative belief systems bring about negative experiences in your life. Whereas, positive thoughts and positive belief systems create positive experiences in your life. It is an uncomfortable truth that your thoughts, feelings and actions create your reality. It is not the excess weight, it is not your financial lack, it is not your husband or your boss that are the root causes of any difficulty, problem or misery in your life. Excess weight, poverty, and inharmonious or stressful relationships are problems in and of themselves but they are also symptoms of a deeper problem. That problem, which is the root cause, lies in your own thinking, your own negative thoughts, words and actions, your own negative belief systems, and emotional wounding that seriously effect and even create your very own reality.

Knowing this, and to use it to your advantage, is to now allow self-reliance and self-responsibility into your life. I actually like the word responsibility for rather than pointing to unpleasant obligations it points to the <u>ability to respond</u>. The ability to respond to the people in your life, the situations in your life, handling those people and situations in a new way. Maybe you will no longer argue back when provoked, but walk away instead. Maybe you will seek another job, or seek a divorce, or see less of your mother or brother. Maybe you will practice forgiveness to those who hurt you, and you will find loving supporting friends instead of ones that use you or drain you. You cease reacting when your buttons are pushed, but look and see the controlling manipulating antics of others stuck in a pattern that demands you get triggered. When you no longer react when you get triggered by their words or actions and instead adopt new, words and actions — self-protecting words and actions, self-validating and self-assured words and actions, you win — you will find a life free from such people and you will find peace, good health and a stable, naturally slim weight.

A little more about beliefs and how they affect your life. Example — Imagine a woman walking down a street. She is two stone overweight. She is thinking to herself — 'I am confident, I am calm, I am peaceful. I accept my size and shape. Sure, I overate last night but that is ok, I am sure it will all balance out as I continue to eat when hungry and stop when full, mistakes are allowed. I am still learning how to stop when full. I am becoming healthier and slimmer every day. I accept myself.' Does she not look graceful, content and maybe even smiling. She looks like life is good to her and she can handle what life gives her. She is in a good frame of mind to accomplish her goals. Now, I would like you to imagine that same woman walking down that same street thinking to herself — 'I don't like how I look today, I am so fat, I'll never lose this excess weight. I hate myself for eating like that last night. I'm so disgusted with my lack of will power.' Spot the difference? Do you think she is empowering herself to achieve her goals? And with these images I would like to emphasise the following point — The thoughts we think and the belief systems we have in our conscious and subconscious minds do indeed greatly affect how we look, feel, walk, talk and be in this world of ours. Only you have control over what you think and believe. So when you think and believe healthy, wealthy and wise thoughts you help create healthy, wealthy, wise results. When you do this you are tackling your problems at the root-cause level.

Kill the roots of a weed and you are rid of it. We can weed out our own negative thoughts and defeatist belief systems in this permanent way too. Thus healing the root cause and the symptoms of that negative root, for good. Compulsive eating, being overweight and addiction to food when full are all surface symptoms or surface weeds of a deeper root cause. As we effectively change what we think about ourselves and our habits, through affirmations; from lack of confidence to confidence, from inharmony to harmony, from berating to encouragement and support, we get rid of the symptom (excess weight) by getting rid of the root causes in our thinking. We heal our addiction by healing our problematic thinking and behaviour that causes the addiction.

## Healing Beautifully

When you are in the process of losing weight this way it is important to become familiar with what you feel being slim will give you. Is it an increase in self-esteem, a beauty or freedom that you feel is lacking in your life now? Do you feel you would be more popular, more able to make new friends? Do you feel you would automatically be more confident and have more energy?

Exercise 1. What would being slim give you?

Get quiet for a while and turn within and ask yourself: What would being slim give me? Think of and write down five qualities that you feel being slim would give you. Five qualities that you feel are somewhat lacking in your life now.

For example:

If I were slim I would be more confident, secure, carefree, more at one with myself and more able to make friends.

Now ask yourself: How else (other than getting slim) can I acquire this quality? List several activities for each quality that would help you experience that quality now, before you get slim.

For example:

In order for me to develop the attribute of confidence (which I think being slim will give me) I can begin acting as if I am confident – I have heard the phrase - Fake it until you make it – it would be a bit of a stretch for me but I can try. Attending night school now, not waiting until I am slim. Learning to swim now, or do Tai Chi for I have also heard that it is by taking action before you are feeling confident that confidence grows. In this way gently challenging myself to step out of my comfort zone regularly. Also thinking about and appreciating all that I have accomplished so far, praising myself rather than being self-critical would all boost my confidence.

In order for me to develop the attribute of being carefree (which I think goes along with being slim) I could start walking along the beach, go cycling, swim and spend time with friends over a lazy lunch. These activities may help me feel more carefree. I could notice my thinking and see what burdensome attitudes or beliefs I have, such as when I go grocery shopping after work I often feel like just doing a bit of window shopping, and taking a stroll but I always ignore it and scurry on home when there is no pressing need for me to do that.

In order for me to make new friends, I could join a support group, evening class or a mother and toddler group and make friends there. I could even start a book club, learn a language or take up Yoga at a local class. Things I've always wanted to do, things I am interested in and therefore meet like-minded folk. When people have the same interests it is easier to become friends. I could invite that nice neighbour round for a coffee and a chat. I could make the effort to keep in contact with old friends. Even with distance between us a phone call can lead to a visit and pleasant day trip or holiday.

Working on developing your own desired qualities, in this way, ensures that the desired quality is allowed permeate your whole being as you do the emotional and practical work that is required to attain that desired quality.

The point I am making is this – Getting slim alone (being slim in and of itself) will not automatically mean that you get the qualities that you think being slim will give you. Focusing on those qualities you associate with being slim, and working with how you can develop these qualities within you now, does allow you to have those qualities regardless of what size and shape you are.

Let us, at this point, explore further the, very often overlooked reality, that being slim, in and of itself, is not a guarantee of confidence, security, love and beauty or any other positive attribute, that any woman struggling with her weight, may feel would automatically emerge if only she were slimmer. One just has to look around to notice quite a few slimmer sisters also lacking in those precious commodities.

The truth is, that whether you are overweight or slim, if, your confidence or sense of security or any other positive attribute is in short supply, you can do something to change that fact. Changing and improving oneself involves a slightly different approach than just losing a few pounds. Losing our excess weight, without doing emotional resolving, does not give us certain positive or desired character traits. It does not make us better or worse people, it is a body size, a simple reflection of what you have or have not eaten.

However, attending classes, reading self-help books, and getting definite about what we want from life and from ourselves, does help us become the woman we want to be, and we can do that, no matter what size or shape we are!

In her book, Fat Is A Feminist Issue, Susie Orbach rightly states that being fat means waiting until you are slim to live. Let's stop waiting and start living now. You have what it takes and you can do it! Take courage and remember life is for you. You are good enough, rich enough, slim enough and young enough now, regardless of appearances, to be out there doing what you want to be doing. So, no more waiting until you are slim to live. Let's start now!

## Power Positive

To be an empowered woman is the natural outcome of healing your issues around food and fatness. In moving toward being a more empowered woman, most women feel the need to redefine and evolve their ideas of power. Their present concepts of power may be of domination, subtle or overt, from boyfriends, parents or work. Domination or victimisation are the negatives we see around us and on TV. Seeing power as quite an ugly topic they avoid it as best they can.

When we cease using food when full as a means of dealing with our feelings and emotional issues, up comes the issue of power, to be looked at, and resolved. Thus, every woman on her healing journey is faced with the task of redefining what power means for her personally. Let us look at what power really is, from a somewhat spiritual standpoint. To be powerful one must have will. Will is thought and action in harmony. Combined if you like. It is essential to have will in order to bring about positive change in one's behaviour and one's life. Will can also be described as determination or ability. And we need it to accomplish anything!

So, in the rubbish bin with domination and being a victim. We aim for power that is empowering for everyone. To get to this positive type of power, we must first, feel those feelings of powerlessness. You might experience feelings of powerlessness if you find yourself doing something that someone else wants you to do, but you do not really want to do it. Uncomfortable though it may be, it is good to feel the pain associated with this sense of powerlessness, for being thus aware of these feelings will encourage you to be more true to your own needs and wants rather than simply continuing to comply with what another wants you to do, when it is not really what you want to do. In other words you are noticing how painful it is to give your power away. Remember, no one can take your power, they can try, but your power is yours to give or keep. By noticing when you feel the pain of powerlessness you are noticing when you are giving your power away, and to whom; and what they ask, say or do to get it. Thus, with this awareness you can learn to react in such a way as to not allow them access to your power. For example: Your mother asks you to repeatedly take care of your father when she goes shopping, when she could ask the neighbour or see about hiring help. A friend constantly asks you to walk her dog, since her hip surgery, but she could easily afford a dog-walker. In these cases you can tell them you are busy, have plans, or are meeting a friend for lunch; you can also suggest they hire help and even recommend a service. They may give you the silent treatment or play the victim in order to manipulate you out of your power and get you, to again, acquiesce into doing what they want you to do regardless of the fact that you really do not want to, but you can stand your ground and again state you can't help out, as you have other plans. Slowly, or even quickly, they lose their grip on you, and you find your life filled with activities you love to do and want to do, helping only the people that you genuinely <u>want</u> to help, and <u>when</u> you want to help. It's on your terms because it is your life! Your life, your time, your power!

## From Powerlessness to Empowerment

In food addiction, the experience of being a compulsive eater often includes the feeling of being out of control or powerless around food. Food is the object of your addiction, the focus of your attention, that which you are in a power-struggle with, to a greater or lesser extent. Food when full gives you the power to suppress your emotions and it demands the heavy price of excess weight and unresolved issues remaining unresolved. Food has been given power. Being a compulsive eater (someone who regularly eats when already physically full) is all about giving food your power. Food has the power to calm your nerves, to sedate almost, and seemingly fill that empty space inside. Binge eating to squash those feelings of powerlessness leaves us even more powerless. Food eaten when full – an inappropriate substitute for real love and real comfort. Truly loving and comforting ourselves entails delayed gratification. We can learn how to give up the instant self-abusive remedy that the binge on food affords us and know we can feel the uncomfortable feelings; and in so doing, enable them to pass. We can bear the momentary emotional discomfort and hold out for the passing of that emotional discomfort. In issues of power, we must feel our powerlessness in order to be shown how to deal with our powerlessness.

On the other hand, of course, we can stuff those uncomfortable feelings of powerlessness down like this, thinking – Oh yes, food has all the power and once the binge has started there is no stopping you. The diet begins tomorrow. More and more you eat. Maybe you will stop at the next biscuit, or sandwich, or bowl of cereal. Who knows? But you do know something – You are out of control. I know, I was once there.

This is a painful experience and thankfully one that can be healed. The healing starts with feeling those painful feelings of powerlessness for it is that pain that fuels the will, the will and determination to take action and ensure that it never happens again. When we have will, we have power. This is positive power remember.

## Powerlessness

Powerlessness is doing what another wants when it is in direct violation of what you wish; and this results in feelings of powerlessness and pain. Always be aware that you are responsible for the decisions you make. Deeply consider and trust your own gut-instincts. Think ahead and consider the outcome of each choice, to help you determine what choice is best. This could even be a simple thing such as – Do I really want to babysit on Saturday? Or as complex as – Do I want a home birth?

However, if you have forsaken your own gut instincts and done what another wanted instead of what you wanted, then you will no doubt be feeling powerless and possibly a tad guilty. This is natural guilt, just to remind you not to do that again.

Take heart all is not lost. You will learn far more from a mistake than you ever will from a success! Through feeling these feelings of powerlessness you are allowing them to integrate and thus providing yourself with the energy that fuels your intentions and will. You then have the power and courage to accomplish and get the results you truly know are right for you in all areas of life. Thus you are empowered. Your intention and will thus are energy filled.

However through running away from feelings by eating when full thus suppressing them we are food addicts. It takes a lot of energy to suppress a feeling so our energy gets depleted, leaving us with less energy to fuel our intentions and will. We have less power to accomplish and try. Thus we remain stuck, with little power to change. Suppressing our feelings of powerlessness leaves intention and will with little energy and we end up feeling dissatisfied.

**A quick reminder**

You may ask – How do I know when I am suppressing my feelings? This is a good question, and as far as food addiction is concerned, the answer is simple. Every time you eat when you are not physically hungry, you are suppressing something.

Refrain from eating until you are actually physically hungry again. This will help you become more aware of what exactly, it is, that you are suppressing. In the meantime, ask yourself –

What feeling is this? How does my body feel? What's this all about? And lastly ask yourself – What do I truly want from this situation? This all helps you to contact and stay with those feelings which you were previously stuffing down with food. It bears repeating – Allow yourself to feel and experience these feelings to the full. This alone will enable you to overcome your eating disorder.

Small steps empower you to move from being afraid of the future to aspiring to the future you desire. You may change from doing what others want you to do, when it is not what you want to do, to doing what you want to do, even if others are miffed. You also give others the freedom to do as they wish without allowing them to manipulate you or harm you or your loved ones, in any way. In other words, you are in the powerful position of knowing what you feel and what you want from any given situation. You may even watch someone while they are talking to you, trying their best, overtly or covertly, manipulate you into doing things their way – and you still find the right thing for you to say or do to get what you truly want from the situation, even if it sometimes means completely walking away. You are in effect saying – Okay, that is your opinion and you are entitled to it. However, I am the authority over what I do and I choose to do this, even if you object.

You do not harm anyone and you refuse to allow yourself or those you love to be manipulated by convention and mediocrity. You move from, running away from reality to taking responsibility for and actively creating the reality you want. For through feeling your feelings you now have energy filled intention and will. This is power positive.

Affirm – It is safe for me to be an empowered woman. I now get what I truly desire in life. Through my positive and powerful thoughts, words and actions I am free, I am healthy, I am empowered, prosperous and fulfilled.

**To waist or not to waste**

No, I have not spelt it wrong! The printers have not made an error. And forgive me Shakespeare but this is a very accurate pun on several concepts which seem to be all mixed up within society in general as regards food and wastage. Let us get one thing straight, being obese does not stop world hunger. Let me explain:

How many of us were encouraged to eat that extra spoonful beyond our natural physical fullness whilst being reminded of some hungry child somewhere? Well, there was one thing for sure, if this was your experience, you were not that starving child, no you were its Western counterpart, the child whose mother was not listening when you said 'No thanks Mum. I am full!' By thus ignoring your exclamations of fullness and actively overriding your body's natural and accurate fullness signals, your mother set the blueprint for the future overriding of your own fullness signals by none other than yourself. So many of us have experienced this, and we also got the message that we must trust some outer authority to tell us what our stomachs have been trying to tell us all along – what and when to eat! A paving stone in the pathway towards food addiction.

In truth those hunger an fullness signals can be listened to by children and parents alike. Children, babies and toddlers all automatically know, listen to and trust what their stomachs are telling them and in turn will tell you when they are hungry. They will express what they want to eat too. When listened to and respected by their parents the child grows up feeling supported and trusting their own hunger and fullness sensations and will never have an eating disorder. The child's inner knowing has be validated allowing a natural, healthy and enjoyable relationship to food be established as nature intended.

How then do we tackle the very real problem of wastage? The idea of wasting as little as possible is very important to all of us as individuals and on a global scale. The more we can get our thinking straight on this issue the better for all of us. A lot of you are very conscious of the problem of wasting food and rightly so. However if that concern causes you to stuff food into your already full stomach or demand empty plats at mealtimes, you are hardly responding to your own hunger and fullness signals appropriately, nor respecting your loved ones' ability to know when they are full. In fact, you are actively encouraging within them a lack of trust in their own ability to recognise and act appropriately on their own sensations of physical fullness. If you find yourself doing this, it is probably just a reflection of your own dysfunctional upbringing around food. So do not be too hard on yourself, recognise your actions, forgive yourself and resolve to change. If you do not, you could be contributing to your own child's eating disorder.

Women often acknowledge the urge to tell others to 'eat up' when they are dining in company, and that company is leaving food on their plate simply because they have eaten enough and are physically full. It is good to notice these urges and allow others the space to know and trust their own inner cues of physical fullness, be those people your husband, your children or your dinner guests.

It is hard to imagine that this stems from ideas of wanting to prevent wastage. Considering that it is a far greater waste to abuse yourself or your children by ignoring the importance of the 'I am full' signal, which is there, after all, for a very good reason – to tell you when it is time to stop eating and allow the food already in the stomach to be digested, absorbed, converted into energy and used to renew this intricate, miraculous organism known as the human body.

Let us no longer ignore, or encourage others to ignore these subtle inner cues. Instead, let us consider these gentle signals as messages of inner wisdom that are accompanying us throughout life and guiding us to greater health and wellbeing than we have ever known.

**Your stomach is the best dietitian in town!**
It is logical, effective and practical to look to your own stomach, and the sensations emanating from it, for guidance as to your food intake. This amazing organ, will offer you some of the most

valuable solutions to your weight and eating problems. All you have to do is listen to its signals and trust them. Let us consider two important facts. (1) This organ is the one most connected with food due to the fact that its sole purpose is to digest it! (2) This organ is intimately connected to you, being located right inside your body!

So, your stomach is a bridge if you like, a bridge between you and food. It contains the food you eat, therefore it is aware of your food intake, for when it is full, it gently prompts you to stop eating. It is a master of digestion and organises that digested food into energy that empowers you to move. With the nutrients, your muscles and tissues are replenished and cells renewed, any excess food or fuel becomes excess weight. In short, food, and your stomach with all its automatic goings on – keeps you alive!

Your stomach sends you hunger signals when it needs more fuel (food) for the body to function. Fuel which is turned into energy. Obviously if you ignore it's stop the input of fuel signal, which comes in the form of the fullness sensation and give it too much fuel, that extra fuel is what gets turned into fat. Therefore, the food that you eat whilst ignoring your stomach's fullness sensations, is not used as energy or replenishment, it is stored as fat cells in your body.

So, is this the alternative guide to the diet sheet? Yes! Your stomach is going to take over the very important job of helping you with, not only the amount of food you eat, but also the types of food you eat. This is your very own, very accurate, very professional and knowledgeable inner dietitian.

This is all too simple, I hear you cry. If it was this simple then why haven't we been doing it all along? Well, we were not allowed to do it all along. In our young lives we were taught not to trust our appetite and the signals sent from the stomach through words like – You can't possibly be hungry again! Or – You are eating again! You are always eating! Wait until dinner time! You've just eaten! Oh that will be so bad for you! You'll gain pounds! Eat up! Finish everything on your plate! No sweets before dinner! Your upset, here have a chocolate bar! After all the time I spent cooking and now you won't eat! You can't possibly be full! Eat and be strong! You will eat what I give you! You have to eat meat!

We never stopped to think that whomever taught us to finish everything on our plates even though we were full, was wrong. However it is true, these well-meaning people who did their best, were labouring under a misconception - the misconception that to encourage someone to eat beyond physical fullness was a good idea. The inaccuracies of what they taught us are what we are left with today. Sometimes it is painful for us, even as adults, to realise that our parents are only human and are capable of making mistakes. Do not be surprised at such feelings when you notice their eating patterns and attitudes about weight and food as you adopt these new ideas and are around them.

Why ask a diet sheet what defines an excess amount of food for you when that fluctuates from day to day and is influenced by several variables? These variables include what you ate previously, how long it has been since you last ate, whether you were doing physical work regularly or not, what amount of energy you have recently expended and whether or not you recently used food to suppress feelings. You already have a built-in mechanism, which can tell you all you need to know in order to lose weight and maintain that weight loss effortlessly, through the very basic hunger and fullness sensations. Your stomach is a very accurate guide. An expert to advise you on the ideal food intake for your body at any given moment in time. Remember, it's job is to digest your food and it is located right inside you. Thus it knows what you had for lunch today and yesterday, and whether or not you need to eat right now.

The stomach also allows the body to automatically absorb any excess weight that has been accumulated through overeating when you tune into what it is telling you by way of the hunger and fullness sensations. It is you own best dietitian, so make an appointment for regular consultations – they are free!

## Accomplishing your goal

A relaxed attitude toward anything you try to attain always helps. They say you cannot have something until you do not need it. Taking the neediness out of the equation, taking the neediness out of wanting your ideal weight is always a good idea. Develop a faith that the healthy, slim body you desire is coming to you in a wonderful way as you follow our food-addiction-busting guidelines!

## Thoughts, words and actions produce results

Acknowledging that your thoughts, words and actions not only produce results, but also actually create your reality, entails taking complete responsibility for your own life. This can be a bit tricky if you are an addict, considering that addiction is all about running away from that dreaded reality. However, it is essential that we face our present reality, our fears and learn how to function as effectively as possible whilst feeling our feelings.

Once you grasp this metaphysical truth you are then in a position to consciously change the reality you have created (albeit unconsciously) into a new one. Your power tools to accomplish this are your own thoughts, words and actions, a simple, magic success formula. Change what you think, change what you say both to yourself and others, change what you do, and the result is that you change your outer reality in a permanent way.

Just as re-landscaping a garden requires tools, spades, seeds etc., to change our thoughts we must also use the tools of affirmations (our words) with persistence. Visualisations are also powerful tools to help us psychologically prepare for what we are affirming and help us believe it will indeed come to us.

Your affirmations act as the spade digging into the subconscious mind and uprooting those negative thought weeds so that they can be discarded and replaced with positive thought, flower seeds, that will grow and bloom. Visualising daily what you wish your world was like, is akin to bulbs pushing up through the soil at the appointed time and blossoming forth as visible flowers of positive feelings and good results.

Persistence like sunshine enables growth and ripening of fruit. The satisfaction of when buds open to reveal their colour and we see the outer results of all that inner work. For you the affirmation 'I am slim' has come true, along with a few other heartfelt desires.

Soil soaking up refreshing rain is you soaking up positivity. Positive thoughts, mental pictures and positive feelings concerning the attainment of your goal, being absorbed by mind, body and soul, form a new perspective and a new positive reality after their kind. Where you are now, is fertile soil indeed, for such accomplishments. So you get the idea, and I appreciate you might be thinking - Enough with the gardening metaphor already, let's crack on with the issue at hand.

## But it's not working – I haven't lost any weight yet!

If you find yourself thinking this then stop for a moment and consider this issue further. Firstly, consider what it takes to lose weight this way. Remind yourself of the three main guidelines at the beginning of this book. These are the keys which enable us to automatically find and maintain our own natural weight.

Have a look at the following questions. Answer - Yes - to these questions and you have the definition of a <u>recovered</u> compulsive eater (one who regularly stops when full).

(a)     Am I eating when physically hungry and stopping when physically full 100% of the time?

(b)     Can I say I accept my size and shape exactly as it is right now?

(c)     Am I pinpointing and resolving my emotional issues rather than 'stuffing them down' with food when full?

If your answer is - Yes - to all of these questions then you are either already at your ideal weight and completely healed of any addiction to food when full, or you have completed the first stage of healing – that is, you have conquered your tendencies toward addiction but still carry the excess weight. Weight loss is, however, assured as you continue to follow those guidelines. Have faith in yourself and this logical method that works. The permanent loss of excess weight is the inevitable result in the near future for all of you.

If your answer to all these questions is – No – then you are just starting on your road towards permanent weight loss, and no weight loss is possible until you are answering – Yes – to all three questions. If your answer is – No – to (a) and (c) then you are still a food addict, for you are still using food to distance yourself from your uncomfortable feelings by eating when not physically hungry. The remedy is the 'Am I Hungry ? Table previously mentioned.

**Questions and Answers**

Q. What stands between you and your goal?

A. Between you and where you want to be (your goal) are psychological blocks. Reaching your goal depends greatly on the dissolving of those blocks. Do remember a change of focus can be a great help here. Instead of focusing on all that is blocking your progress, persistently focus on the desired result, preferably for a few minutes nightly before sleep or first thing in the morning. A vision board or note book with pictures representing your desired goal can help.

Q. What stops us from getting slim?

A. Subconscious fears of being slim can come in the form of hidden, negative, assumptions that we have made about being slim. Remember, you are not consciously aware of the associations that your subconscious mind has made about being slim. Being slim equals unwanted advances, feeling too vulnerable, or fears of being promiscuous are common subconscious fears.

Q. How do I deal with these fears and psychological blocks?

A. Visualisation and affirmation. The previous fat/slim visualisation can help unearth these issues so you can be aware of them, address and heal them. Through visualisation you open a doorway to what lies in your subconscious mind and thus become aware of any fearful thoughts about being slim. (Try the visualisations in Susie Orbach's book Fat Is A Feminist Issue.) Once you realise what exactly it is that frightens you about being slim, you can resolve your fears by considering how you would face them if they happened in reality, and reassure yourself that you can indeed deal with your fears effectively.

As I mentioned earlier, what often emerges, for women on this weight loss journey of introspection and healing, is a fear of being exposed to unwanted advances and that they would be unable to protect themselves if they are the slim attractive woman. Or they feel they might become promiscuous because they have the opportunity to sleep around due to their slim figure. The associations here are – Slim means getting unwanted advances, and slim means sleeping around. After uncovering these associations, we can challenge them. Are they really true? Is every slim woman unable to deal with unwanted advances? Is every slim woman promiscuous? Is every fat woman safe from unwanted advances and celibate or unerringly faithful? What is required here is a close look at the issues of unwanted advances and sleeping around.

Ask yourself – How do I handle unwanted advances? How else could I protect myself? How many sexual partners is too many? Are there different standards for men and for women in that area?

Do reassure yourself that you can learn how to deal with these issues successfully. Talk about them with your friends, a therapist, or support group. That may help you find the resolving of these issues that will allow you to be slim, safe and free.

Affirm – I am safe. I am secure. I am protected. I can easily protect myself in any situation.

If you are still unsure then you could resolve to attend an assertiveness workshop or self-defence class.

As for the issue of being promiscuous when slim again challenge your assumptions, ask yourself – Are all slim women promiscuous, simply because they are slim? No. So, promiscuity is not an attribute of slimness. Are fat women never promiscuous? Is it simply impossible for a fat woman to be promiscuous simply due to her size? Of course not! Our body size does not dictate our sexual activities. It is, in truth the responsibility of each individual woman, fat or slim, to decide on her own sexual activity.

What would help here is a good think about the issue of sexuality and what it means to you personally. Ask yourself what qualities you would like in a partner and if you want to have more than one partner. Thus by asking yourself these question, you confront the issue head on, you resolve the issue, it is out in the open so to speak and not just in the unconscious realm of - I'm fat, I'm celibate or I'm slim and I'm promiscuous.

In this way, through pondering the issues at hand, you automatically dissolve the psychological block of fear around the issues of sleeping around and unwanted advances. Promiscuity and unwanted advances may not be your issues. However, it is important to be aware of what your own personal issues are. You can pinpoint your issues by looking at the areas of your life that you feel are problematic, such as your relationship with your mother, or your career. Also, anywhere you have a knee-jerk reaction is a good place to find unresolved emotional stuff to work on.

Ask yourself – How does this situation leave me feeling? Thus you have pinpointed your emotional issue. Also ask – What am I afraid will happen in this situation? Once you know what you are afraid of you can handle your fear. Ask yourself – Is this fear rational or irrational? How can I best handle this fear? Are there steps I can take to protect myself? Is it possible that this thing I am afraid of may never actually happen? And even if it did I could handle it. How can I avoid it happening? You open up a lot of choices for solutions when you step back and question or confront your fears. You can transform your fears into excitement, where the worst does not happen. And you do not let fear prevent you trying something you wanted to try. Fear can paralyse, but if you step back and look at it, feeling neutral, you can make wise choices. This can help you overcome those previously hidden fears around being the slim attractive woman and help you become the person you want to be regardless of your body size.

Whilst your thought associations about what it means to be fat and what it means to be slim, still remain in the depths of your subconscious mind they will prove to be psychological blocks between you and healthy slimness. So, do the previously mentioned fat/slim visualisation at least once a week. You can ask a friend to read the one in this book or the one from Fat Is a Feminist Issue, or you can record it and play it back when you need to as required. This will help you familiarise yourself with the fears that lie in your subconscious mind; and knowing your own personal fears is not only extremely useful, but very necessary in the process of becoming permanently slim.

Q. What else stops us from being slim?

A. Not having the healthy, alternative ways of dealing with life and its challenges. To eat when not physically hungry is a means by which you suppress your unresolved feelings and emotional issues. Suppression as a means of coping, is, and has proven itself to be ineffective, leaving you overweight, with unresolved emotional issues and an eating disorder. In order to give up one means of coping (the ineffective one) we must find a replacement means that is better and more appropriate. The previously mentioned - Am I hungry? Table, plus the various tools and ideas throughout this book help us find each healthier more effective replacement means of dealing with life, it's challenges and all the feelings and emotional issues involved.

Q. What else can help us heal our eating habit?

A. Discovering what purpose your excess weight is serving.

Q. How do I do that?

A. The purpose your excess weight is serving is often subconscious and may need a visualisation to uncover. While visualising yourself at the larger size, and then at the smaller size, ask yourself – If my excess weight had a voice what would it say to (my mother, spouse, boss etc)? This will give you some insight into what issues are there, and what your excess weight (like a separate entity) is trying to do on your behalf. The thing is, that a part of you believes that if you give up the excess weight you also give up this ally or helper. You need to ponder how else you can convey what the 'excess weight' is conveying. It could be saying for example, to your boss – Hey, notice me I deserve a raise! So, you may want to explore the idea of approaching him yourself and asking for a raise, or seriously seeking better paid employment even though it seems impossible. Being aware of, and processing this situation and its associated feelings, is part of what giving up compulsively eating over it entails.

**So when in a relaxed meditative state ask yourself:**
How does my excess weight help me out at work, at a party, at home?
What is the positive purpose of my excess weight?
Does my excess weight protect me in some way?
How else can I protect myself?
How does my excess weight help me when I am with my boss, lover, best friend, mother, father, brother and sister?
Take a little time and visualise yourself both fat and slim in the presence of each one of these people in turn and see what comes up for you in the form of thoughts, ideas, insights or even mental pictures. Write down your findings in a private notebook if you wish, and you will be discovering a whole, previously hidden layer to your weight loss dilemma. And this information will help you resolve that dilemma once and for all. For it is finding other ways, through your perspective, your understanding, your words and your actions that you can do the job you unconsciously gave to your excess weight. Did your excess weight even do that job well? Ask yourself: What action or attitude on my part could do that job well and successfully achieve the result I strive for in being overweight?
Q. What makes it difficult to get slim?
A. Self-criticism, guilt, lack of self-acceptance. These three beauties hinder your progress. Face up to them, feel the feelings

associated with them and practice the alternative attitudes of self-acceptance, self-forgiveness and integrity. As you do, you will see the changes within and without.

Q. How do I deal with guilt?

A. Guilt is the feeling that you have done something wrong in a world that is not safe. So the more you can feel safe, notice safety, acknowledge how you can indeed keep yourself and your loved ones safe, the easier it is to drop guilt, and alive an enjoyable life.

Acknowledge that you have done nothing wrong; you have always acted to the best of your ability given the person you were at that time in your life. Now forgive yourself if you feel you have done something wrong, resolve to never do that again; thus purging yourself of the mistakes of the past, learning a valuable lesson and allowing yourself to become a wiser person as a result. Self-forgiveness is a daily practice that can easily be done. I personally love the forgiveness prayers of healer Howard Wills who you can find on You Tube or at www.howardwills.com

Q. How to deal with self-criticism?

A. Again self-forgiveness helps a lot. Lighten up on yourself and focus on your achievements and good points. When you notice yourself being critical, think of something to praise instead, count your blessings, acknowledge your irritation or anger towards yourself and know that it is harmful and needs to be dropped, transmuted and transformed into healthy self-love as you work on healing what needs to be healed and changing what needs to be changed. A constant barrage of self-criticism does not help you heal and change. Forgive yourself, the situation, your actions, know you can change and the odd slip up can be forgiven, learned from and moved on from.

Q. What is a psychological block?

A. A psychological block is a belief that is preventing you from doing what you want to do. It can be conscious or subconscious. An example of a conscious psychological block would be – I want to enrol in an evening class but feel fearful every time I think about taking a step in that direction. Or – I want to go to the cinema tonight but all my friends are busy and I won't go alone for fear of feeling uncomfortable. I just don't believe that a woman should go out alone. Or – I think about starting my own business and I immediately think I can't do it, it will be too difficult, something will go wrong.

These thoughts may seem valid enough but they are preventing you from doing what you want to do. Your fearful thoughts and beliefs leave no room for thoughts, beliefs and actions that ensure your safety. Look closely and see if your beliefs are preventing you from being out there living life and enjoying yourself.

It can, of course, be more complicated than that. A long-standing problem such as excess weight could have many psychological blocks between you and accomplishing freedom from that problem. Deep-seated negative thought patterns and belief systems such as – I am not good enough. I do not want to be slim because slim women are shallow and cold. I fail at everything. My mother was fat and I am just like her. What's the use? I can't maintain weight loss. I don't deserve a slim body.

All these negative thoughts provide us with a brick wall of resistance, which must be addressed before we can truly improve our quality of life and achieve our goal successfully. Again you may not be consciously aware of these negative thoughts but affirmations and the fat/slim visualisation will help you uncover them.

Q. How can positive thoughts dissolve psychological blocks?

A. Since psychological blocks are created by negative or self-defeating beliefs, positive thoughts and beliefs have the power to cancel out or weaken the effect of those negative beliefs. Just as negative thoughts create blocks, positive thoughts dissolve them, creating a path to your goal. Turn any negative, self-defeating thought into its positive opposite and you have the power to reverse the effects of that negative thought.

Q. Why is it so important for us to feel our feelings?

A. Feeling our feelings puts us in contact with a deeper part of ourselves – our real needs. Real needs, that when fulfilled really make life worth living. Our feelings point us towards those real needs. Only when we are in contact with our needs can we know and begin to meet those needs appropriately, instead of suppressing them by eating when full. We can only meet our needs appropriately when we are truly in touch with our feelings. Meeting our needs appropriately leads to greater satisfaction than we have ever known before, giving us a stronger sense of self too.

Q. When will I lose the excess weight?
A. When you are eating when hungry and stopping when full 100% of the time. Resolving the emotional issues rather than suppressing them with food when full. And when you have high self-acceptance you will enjoy your new, slim-self.

Q. What makes an addict?
A. Lack and negativity play their part in causing addiction. If you have come from a dysfunctional family, if you have suffered childhood abuse, then you probably have some powerful feelings that are quite painful to experience. The temptation is to suppress them. If you give in to this temptation, you are an addict. Feeling the feelings, resolving the emotional issues that drives you to be an addict is the key to recovery. Developing a belief in abundance and a positive attitude help in the process of healing addiction.

Q. What is addicted behaviour?
A. It is behaviour that enables us to avoid / suppress our feelings and emotional issues as opposed to behaviour that enables us to feel our feelings, integrate our feelings and nurture oursleves.

Q. Isn't it because the food tastes so good that I can't stop eating it?
A. It is truly a pleasure to enjoy the wonderful and incredibly varied tastes food has to offer. These pleasurable taste sensations can only be truly enjoyed when you are physically hungry. For eating done when you are already physically full is certainly not pleasurable. As we now know there is only one

thing that drives us to eat when full and that is our unresolved emotional stuff.

Q. What does working on myself involve?

A. It involves a willingness to look at yourself and your life without judgement but with a willingness to change. It usually means facing your fears. Looking at your unresolved emotional issues and discovering how to resolve them. Learning to accept and like yourself as you are before you become the person you want to be, and have the life you want to have. Enjoying where you are and respecting who you are now. Doing whatever you can with the situation in which you now find yourself.

Working on yourself also involves asking for help. Possibly seeing a therapist or healer. Joining a support group or a further education class. Reading or studying self-help books and applying the principles therein, to your day to day life. This could be doing a visualisation or some written exercise, speaking aloud some affirmation in private or simply adopting a more positive outlook on life. This will all influence your life for the better and it is called working on yourself.

Q. What do I do if I am flooded with negative experiences?

A. It is taking a lot longer that you wanted, or you just feel that you are not getting a handle on it. Maybe the results you want are just not materialising. If this is your experience then do not despair. If you are overcoming an eating disorder, and it is just one negative experience after another, here are some ideas to help: Remember it sometimes gets worse before it gets better.

Ask yourself: Am I criticising myself or beating myself up about this rather than focusing on my accomplishments no matter how small or trivial they may seem to be?

Be very aware when you answer this question, for most of you are busy overriding your accomplishments and finding great ways to invalidate your achievements. Most women are accomplishing far more than they are giving themselves credit for. It is quite a skill to be able to breathe deeply, and acknowledge that you are doing just fine. Okay, maybe your progress is slower than you want. Maybe even frustratingly so. Do not worry. It is certainly not a sign of failure. It definitely is a sign that you have more psychological blocks to work through, more skills to learn and more painful issues to resolve. Maybe you need to develop more patience or persistence.

Ask yourself: How can I lighten up on myself about this?

Know that simply more inner work is required if the desired outer results have not yet materialised. Maybe a negative, painful pattern throughout your life needs to be seen and acknowledged. So, become quiet, relax your mind and quiet your emotions, or, allow a space of peace to be between you and your emotions; close your eyes and ask your higher self, God, the Angels, Source (whatever you believe in) – What is the perfect solution to this issue? Is there anything else I need to know about how to heal this negative pattern, heal my eating disorder, or solve this life issue I am having? Listen out for guidance, it may come immediately or in a few days.

In my own experience, it has always been darkest before the dawn. I gained weight before achieving my own permanent weight loss and complete healing of my eating disorder. Before a new career came to me, I went through some very tough obstacles and series of negative experiences, spanning years, before I broke through those negative experiences and established the career I had long desired, studied for and had worked toward. I must say at this stage there were also positive aspects of my life which brought great joy to me during those years, regardless of the negative experiences and dark hours. My ability to make the best of a bad lot was very useful in my dealing with and overcoming the challenges life was giving me. Also the fact that I was consciously studying and working towards a career I knew I truly loved was tremendously uplifting in itself.

How do you attain lasting improvement in all areas of life?
Evolving as a human being involves awareness of your true self, your feelings, your actions and your surroundings. Work with your attitudes, notice your thoughts and feelings concerning each issue and area of life. Clear out old negative thoughts, doubts and fears about achieving your desired goals. Replace negative beliefs, thoughts and feelings, through daily affirmation and visualisation, with more positive, life-enhancing, confidence building thoughts, beliefs and feelings.
Repeating positive affirmations daily, actively develops positive feelings, integrity and understanding. Taking whatever appropriate action is in line with positive thoughts and feelings,

brings the accomplishment of the desired result. This is very empowering stuff! A positive frame of mind, positive feelings and positive action are all very productive, not only enhancing your chances of achieving your goal, but also enabling you to do so. Whereas a negative frame of mind and negative thoughts, feelings and actions tend to hinder and repel the achievement of that goal. So be very aware of your thoughts and feelings.

**What to do, with what you would love to do?!**
When there is something you would love to do:-
(a)    First acknowledge you want it. Then:
(b)    Write down your plan for achieving it, in a much detail as possible.
(c)    Mentally accept it as possible for you. Say affirmations stating the perfect accomplishment of your goal, until you believe them and you feel that your desired result is possible and probable for you.
(d)    Visualise it
(e)    Work toward it. In other words take action. Follow up on those hunches, bright ideas and inner guidance.
(f)    Persist, be flexible and believe you can succeed.
(g)    And at last, relax and let go emotionally (if it comes it comes, if it doesn't it doesn't). Watch it manifest in its own time and in its own way. It may come in a form different than you expect, but none the less, you have to admit that it is the manifestation of that gaol accomplished. All you have to do is

receive it thankfully and with appreciation for yourself working hand in hand with the universal life force energies of creation.

**Practical Work**

Not being good enough – Can you remember specific instances of feeling not good enough? In the present, do you often have the feeling of not being good enough? Does someone close often leave you feeling that way? Could the problems in your life be the products of a subconscious – I am not good enough, I do not have enough, I do not do enough – thought pattern? If so, can you recall a childhood situation where you did not feel good enough? Did what someone said influence how you felt? In other words did someone make you feel as if you were not good enough? If so, what did they say or do? What was their tone of voice? Does something similar get said to you in present day situations?

Recall any past event in which you felt not good enough. Recall who is present. The feelings and the situation. Now forgive yourself for any wrong you feel you may have done. Forgive the others involved who you feel hurt you or made you feel uncomfortable. See the old unpleasant scene erased, enveloped in light until it is like a clean white board and start to visualise another scene where you are experiencing love and approval from all concerned.

**Money Matters!**

Just like food, money can be an emotionally charged substance. We have embodied it with power, security and other such qualities, which it does not, in fact contain. Issues of money often arise when we are healing our eating habit. Money is important in this money age and materialistic society. None of us can get away from it. And most of us want more of it. It is essential to our basic needs in life such as food, housing and clothing. Also a necessity when it comes to education, recreation, and travel. Enjoyment of life, may even seem to depend on it and to a certain extent does.

These pieces of metal and paper are loaded with emotional stuff. Just like food, we must be aware of our issues around money and resolve them to insure that we do not transfer our unresolved emotional issues on to money, and suddenly become obsessed with money instead of our weight and food. Key obsessive thoughts to watch out for would be – If only I were richer. Echoes of the – If only I were slimmer – routine.

Just as there are differences between your fat-self and your slim-self, it is good to notice any marked differences between your rich-self and poor-self. It is also useful to uncover any subconscious fears around becoming financially free. A slim and healthy body is your birthright, so is financial freedom. Many people associate human qualities, such as security, peace of mind, personal happiness, status and power with what is only paper and metal (or plastic as in a debit card). In and of themselves they cannot provide any of these benefits. All of those qualities mentioned, can of course be developed only by turning within and allowing them to develop from deep within ourselves, regardless of the contents of our purse!

When the Universe / God / Source / Divine Intelligence, or whatever you wish to call it, is recognised as the source of all things tangible and intangible, then it is easier to create money in your life, and from work you love. We all have our own unique talents and abilities. I call them gifts, the things we love to do, God given gifts that prove to be a gift to you because of the enjoyment and prosperity you get from their right use. They are a gift to others because of the needed service you provide. The Creator's gifts, be they in the field of psychology, maths, art or healing, are those things you love doing or are interested in. You were born with the ability to flourish in that field because of your interest and love. They were given to you concerning a Divine Plan, by a bigger power than any of us can comprehend and are meant to be expressed through you. They are always needed, otherwise She would not have given them to you. Do not be like most people who refuse to acknowledge that they could possibly fulfil their hearts desire, or be of real benefit to others. Finding your own gifts and interests, developing your gifts and interests is always possible either in big or small ways at any given moment in time. The truth is that it does not matter who you know, or what you know, how much money you have or what type of education you have. Start now, with who you are now, accept it and take up the challenge of a lifetime (your lifetime) to change what you have now into your heart's desire. You would be surprised what is possible when you are on the right track, flowing with your own intuitive guidance and heartfelt interests. The only person who really fails is the one who does not even try.

If you want to have more money, visualise yourself rich then poor using our fat/slim visualisation but substituting slim for rich and fat for poor, paying attention to your feelings and beliefs about these two states, unearthing the positive of poor and the negative of rich. Resolve to heal the negative of rich and promise yourself to bring with you the positive of poor as you increase your wealth. This can be very enlightening, informative and interesting.

**Keys to financial success**

Recognising that the creative intelligence and energy of the universe is the source of all. What is the creative intelligence of the universe? It is what people refer to a God, Allah, Buddha, Divine Intelligence, Universal Wisdom, the Divine Mother or Divine Substance. It is the ultimate source of all that is tangible and intangible. The source of all, that includes money, food, clothes, ideas, inspiration, opportunities, relationships and guidance.

Connecting with this source can be done through meditation, relaxation, breathwork, prayer or Yoga. Also being aware of and following with courage gut feelings and intuition – literally Source whispering to you.

Experimenting with what is intuitive guidance and what is not. Allowing yourself to get to know what true inner guidance is by taking small steps, small healthy risks, and noticing how they turn out. Accepting an opportunity to travel, take a course or new job for example. Thus developing a trust in this new-found friend, your intuition which emerges in your daily activities, although more noticeably during times of relaxation and meditation. An example of this would be – You get the idea to leave some leaflets advertising your workshop in a local community centre. You follow up on the idea. You go to that community centre and ask permission to pin your notice on their board. They say yes, you are pleased and a few days later you get a call from someone who saw your leaflet there and wishes to attend your workshop.

Trust in the Source and your connection with the Source. This comes automatically as you practice and gain the results you desire by working with your intuition. You can develop your trust by taking more and bigger healthy risks, with your increasing confidence.

Visualise your way to financial success. It is said that if you can hold it in your mind, you can have it in your life. So be aware of what it is that you are picturing. Hold in your mind pictures of yourself as slim, prosperous, healthy, joyful, successful, compassionate and wise. Visualise your plans and visualise them in detail. Remember goodness lies in the details.

Affirm that you do deserve the best in life. It is okay for you to have the best. Many of us were taught as children by scolding parents 'You don't deserve it!' concerning some good thing we wanted, and even shockingly 'You deserved it!' concerning a beating. This can all be forgiven and healed.

Know that it is ideas which are acted upon, and persistence in doing what you love, that creates lasting prosperity and happiness with that prosperity and wealth.

Tithe a tenth of your income. This literally means, give a tenth of your financial income to whomever is giving you spiritual help and inspiration before you start to spend any of that particular sum of money – a pay check for example. Tithing is a Universal or Metaphysical Law. It is said the number 10 is the magic number of increase and overflowing, through giving a tenth of your financial income to the person or organisation that you feel is giving you spiritual inspiration, you are making room to receive an increased amount of what you have given away – money. Through giving to your inspiration point, you are connecting in a very real way to the universal inspiration point – the source of all wealth – Spirit or Source Energy. Thus you are affirming and acknowledging with your own money the source of all money – God, Love, The Divine Mother, Source (whatever you feel comfortable calling It). Quite a business connection!

Maybe you are resisting the idea of giving away a tenth of your income. I am not surprised. It is a wise thing to question and speculate before making any financial decision. What I would say to you is this – Read a Catherine Ponder book called The Dynamic Laws of Prosperity (it is also free as a You Tube audio now I believe), specifically chapter 10 which is on tithing. You will never look back! I personally have been tithing since I was

27 and I cannot fault it. It continues to give me a sense of abundance and security that nothing else ever has.

It could be a church, an individual involved in spiritual healing or an organisation such as AA that is giving you comfort and support. The important thing is to give your tithe where you are receiving that spiritual inspiration. The practice of tithing gives you a sense of financial wealth and security, regardless of your income. Tithing not only creates a vacuum, which draws more money into it, but also seems to stretch the other nine tenths further, so financial needs are met. Most importantly, in my experience, acknowledging God / Source by tithing brings an absence of money worries. Or if there are worries, I am more able to handle them. Most people try tithing when they feel they have nothing to lose. When I started tithing I soon realised it was the best financial decision I had ever made, and I still enjoy tithing, reaping the rewards of this ancient and true practice.

**Wealthy Women**

Just as with power, money has somewhat of a bad reputation and just like food it is seen as overindulgent to have a lot. Especially for women, to be financially free is often an issue; but let us remember that money itself is neutral. It is the purpose to which money is put that determines whether it is positive or negative. Money and power are often mistakenly linked. Just like our attitudes about power need to be allowed to evolve so do our attitudes about money. We may have to look closely at our ideas about money before we can be able to use the amount we have effectively and in ways which meet our needs appropriately. Affirm often – There is always enough. This is a powerful thought!

**Affirmation:** Through people and circumstances my prosperity flows, but its source is Infinite. And that Infinite Source guides, prospers and directs my life. I am connected to that true source of all that is, and it nourishes and supplies my every need. For this I am grateful.

**Back to the body – Think slim!**
Regard what you have, as if, it is already what you want. Regard the body you have now, as if, it is the body you want. In other words, act as if you have already achieved your goal. Act as if you are already slim and full of self-acceptance or confidence or whatever it is you feel being slim will give you. You can do this anywhere. While you are waiting for the bus, having lunch or making a pot of tea. Just casually say to yourself – 'Right, I am now the size I have always wanted to be.' And notice how you feel. Keep this thought going through your mind for as long as you can and as often as you can until you actually do become your slim-self. Thus you are mentally preparing yourself for when you really are slim.

Try this visualisation when you are relaxing at home. Perhaps get a friend to read it aloud for you, or record it, leaving a few minutes between each sentence in order for you to picture the scene, and feel the feelings coming up. You can do it right now in fact. Breathe deeply a few times and relax your body and mind deeper and deeper with each exhale. About 10 – 15 long slow deep breaths should do it. Good. Notice if you are holding tension in any part of your body. If so, mentally say 'Relax' to those muscles.

If you are holding on to any worry or concern ask God / The Universe / Saints or Angels or whatever you believe in, to help you release it and let it go. See yourself handing it over to that higher, helpful power and now you are free and relaxed in the knowledge that your concerns are being resolved in perfect ways, easily and in peace, and you can do your visualisation.

**Visualisation**

Say to yourself: I am now my desired weight… I am now perfectly slim… And visualise yourself in an imaginary scene as being the weight you want to be. How do you feel…? What are you doing now that you are your ideal weight…? Visualise your surroundings in as much detail as possible. Are you in a park, at work, at home or a party…? Who is there and how do you feel about these people…? How are they reacting to the slim you…? Notice the feelings being slim gives you… What do you think about the world, as a slim person…? How do you interact with others now you are slim…? How are you around food, relaxed or tense…? How do you feel about your marital status now you are your ideal weight…? What are the main positives about being slim…? What are the negatives in being slim…?

Now I would like you to imagine you are gaining a large amount of weight in the same situation… Notice the differences in what you are wearing, how you feel, and how you are acting and reacting to the others there, now that you are at a very large size (much bigger than you have ever been before)… Be aware of both the positive and negative aspects of being large. Now slowly let the scene fade and open your eyes, stretch your body gently and jot down in your notebook your thoughts and ideas that emerged from that visualisation.

Take special interest in the differences between your fat and slim self and know these are the areas you will be working on at the larger size, for in so doing, you will be able to look at and resolve the negative associations of being slim before you actually become slim. This emotional pinpointing and resolving, further empowers you, by enabling you to see the emotional details and intricacies of allowing your slim-self emerge and become a permanent reality.

## Preparation for your slim self

For a certain amount of time each day, say to yourself – 'Right, I am now slim. I have reached my ideal weight.' I suggest you start early. When you wake. Start the day as if you had already achieved your goal. Now that you are slim what would you wear to work? Is there a certain colour or style of clothes that you would now buy yourself, now you are slim. Colours and styles come in all shapes and sizes so I suggest you do actually buy them at your present size to see how they feel, and thus integrate and resolve those feelings about that style and colour now at the larger size. You have this safety net, if you like, of being the larger size while experimenting with the coming reality of your slim-self.

Continuing to 'think slim' consider – how would you start your day? With a jog perhaps? But what if you do not like jogging? Being slim is not an automatic guarantee of liking jogging! However, if you like swimming now you will probably still like swimming when you lose your excess weight, so maybe a swim is in order? Do it now. Do not wait until you are slim to give yourself permission to go for a swim.

There may be big differences in who you are now and who you are slim. For many women there is a marked difference in the way they relate to the world, themselves and their bodies when they are slim. Resolving and dissolving these differences is essential to permanent weight loss and healing your eating habit. Realising you are the controlling power in your life and that and that being fat or slim does not dictate how you behave or what your opinions are in areas such as sexuality, love, health, work, family and emotional well-being. These are complex issues that only you know how to deal with, and we are excavating that innate knowing through these practices.

Your opinions are yours to evolve, develop and even change if you wish, and you do not have to wait until you are slim to do that, nor presume they will they automatically change just because your body size changes. You can start now. It is okay to start now. In fact, it would be a very good idea to start now, don't you think?

As I mentioned before, how you interact with the world is completely up to you. You can have fun being the aware, detached observer experimenting with how you interact with both loved ones and strangers alike. How you feel is important. Only you can know how you feel, in any given situation and what action, if any, you wish to take on those feelings. One thing is sure, your feelings exist and serve an important purpose. The purpose of telling you something of great consequence about every single situation in which you may find yourself. So, do acknowledge your feelings and emotions for what they are – loving guides.

The more you are able to feel your feelings, the more empowered you are to make accurate decisions about what you want to do in your life. Decisions that are in line with your heart-felt desires and goals inevitably lead you to greater happiness and satisfaction. Not without a challenge or two, but ultimately satisfying none the less. Thus you 'fill yourself up' in invisible, meaningful ways.

Also, the more you are able to feel your feelings, the more you are able to heal past traumas, and resolve, previously unresolved, emotional issues. You get that stuck emotional energy unstuck through the ability to feel your previously suppressed emotions. Stopping when full allows previously suppressed emotions and feelings to surface, and if you meet them with the ability, care and willingness to feel those emotions – you heal your habit of eating when full and thus lose excess weight permanently and naturally.

There is one, and only one thing that heals the urge to overeat (or heals any addiction for that matter) and that is, <u>resolving the root cause, the original traumas and their associated feelings.</u> With the permanent resolving of these feelings and emotional issues, which are caused by the original traumatic or unpleasant events, comes the healing of the addiction. Even though the traumatic event happened in the past the residual feelings are with us today unless we healed them, brought them out of suppression, recognised them and felt them in their unpleasant entirety. As you can now fully realise, the experiencing and resolving of emotional issues and feelings has a lot of beneficial spin offs – the healing of trauma, the healing of the cravings, the healing of the automatic response to suppress emotions, and the healing of the symptom - the addiction to food when full and it's resultant excess weight.

We are dealing with three causes and one result, all linked – Cause 1. The traumas of life. Cause 2. The feelings and emotions linked to those traumas. Cause 3. The activity of eating food when full to deal with them. The One Result - excess weight.

Can feelings be hard to resolve? Sometimes – yes. Sometimes – no. What is needed is a therapist, healer, good friend, or a support group that you like and trust; and if you enjoy a good read, all the better, for the variety and quality of excellent self-help books available today is awe-inspiring. With this support and back up you are then empowered to find and incorporate into your life the tools which enable you to grow out of eating when full, or any addiction, and into a rewarding and fulfilling way of life.

## People are our mirrors

An important point to remember is that people are our mirrors. Basically this means that whatever we see in another person is a reflection of something within ourselves. It is a simple truth which can give us many a valuable insight into who we are, and what issues we need to deal with at any given moment in time. An essential aid in personal development. Now this mirror image, may not be an exact replica of what you have going on in your own life; for me personally it took me years to recognise within myself some character traits that I so clearly saw in another. But just like the face you see in the mirror is an inverted image of your own real three dimensional face, the ugly characteristic we see in our fellow human may contain just an inkling or a whisper of similarity to that quality in ourselves. A quality that we wish to avoid acknowledging and maybe even use food when full to avoid being aware of it.

For example: If you see strength or beauty in another you can know that those are qualities you already possess because you were able to see those qualities in the other person. Likewise, should you see unhappiness or pain in another, realise, that you could have some unresolved issues in those areas. Check in with your inner child by just imagining yourself as a child. Ask her if she is unhappy about anything or in pain about something.

Asking yourself these questions will help you acknowledge what is going on under the surface and help you discover any half-suppressed emotional issues waiting to be acknowledged and resolved for good.

So, let's not dismiss the unpleasant character traits we see in others as simply 'their' character traits, and thus worthy of our criticism. Instead we can be secure enough in who we are to accept that the pleasant and unpleasant character traits we see in others are in fact mirror images of the parts of ourselves which we may or may not like. Those faults we are prone to highlighting and criticising as the other persons defect, is in fact the very part of ourselves which we have been running away from and have projected onto that person. Acknowledging this fact, we can ask ourselves – 'Well, do I have this annoying habit or character trait which I see so clearly in Mr. X?' We see a glimmer of our own incomplete and imperfect selves! So, rather than blame ourselves or others, we simply take responsibility and work towards changing. We can embrace as our own, this previously hidden 'imperfection' and set about righting it, in whatever way seems best.

Both self-forgiveness and forgiving others is very useful in this sort of situation and in personal growth in general. Increased awareness of our own thoughts, actions and reactions is also helpful. Thus we polish and perfect, refine and positively alter the parts of ourselves which we do not like and were even suppressing. We enable ourselves to become the people we want to be and enjoy the freedom of a less critical attitude toward our fellow human beings and ourselves, knowing we are not only mirror images of one other but also one with each other, and discovering what we can do to heal ourselves and our planet, may just be the most important task at hand.

## Who is in the driving seat?

Let me point out at this stage that life brings up both pleasant and unpleasant feelings. What is important to remember is this: How we deal with these feelings makes us either a person with a problem around food, or a person with a healthy, non-addicted relationship to food. As you know, a compulsive eater uses food to suppress those feelings by eating when not even physically hungry. A recovered compulsive eater, or a person with a healthy relationship to food, allows herself to feel and integrate her own feelings, taking healthy action when appropriate. By knowing and respecting her own feelings, and acting in a life-enhancing, positive, healthy way she is in alignment with her own personal value system of what she wants to be doing with herself, her time and her life. For example gardening if she enjoys gardening, painting if she enjoys painting, studying art if she loves art etc. She thus is approaching her life from a more empowered angle than the compulsive-eater that she was. She is now a victor, she overcomes opposing circumstances and often leaves behind difficult people. She is the champion of her own life, not a doormat. She is the one in the driving seat!

## Roller-coaster

Women with an eating disorder often express that the 'going right' or 'going wrong' of a day can get reflected in their eating habits. For example: something happens in the morning, it brings up some unpleasant feelings. The compulsive eater, eats to 'stuff down' those feelings, without ever exploring or resolving them, thus setting herself off on a roller-coaster of overeating for the rest of the day.

What can she do to keep off that sickening roller-coaster? Well, quite a lot really! Suppose you found yourself experiencing some uncomfortable feelings, early in your day. Let's consider the step-by-step formula that you can bring into operation at this moment in time:

1. Acknowledge the feelings and say to yourself something like: Okay, I know I do not like experiencing this feeling but I would like to explore it a little, to see if I can resolve it once and for all.

2. Notice if you have the craving to eat. If you do then ask yourself – Am I physically hungry? If the answer is - 'No, I am not physically hungry, I am full' then we can go about the business of finding the healthy alternative to suppressing our feelings with food when full. This requires relaxing, thinking and focusing.

3. Acknowledge that you can always use food when full in order to stuff those feelings down. Also acknowledge that you are dissatisfied with that old method, and day by day you are becoming more and more willing to find a healthy alternative.

When we are physically full and we do not eat, even though we may have a craving to do so, we are actually allowing ourselves to experience our previously suppressed feelings more fully. Just being aware of this dynamic is important.

4.     Physically relax and ask yourself: What feeling is this? What words can best describe what I am experiencing?

5.     Once you are aware of what this feeling is, you can simply ask yourself: Given the fact I feel this way what would I like to do now?

6.     If you have a favourite uplifting affirmation or quote, a favourite line of poetry or positive saying then this could be an appropriate time to repeat it either aloud or to yourself.

Notice your surroundings and the situation you are in. How do you feel about this situation and these surroundings? Who is around you at this moment? Has something just happened to upset you, at work or at home, in the shops or in a recent conversation? Is this a long-standing dilemma? What small steps can you take, right now, to help you feel more at ease about this situation or problem? How about a change in the way you perceive this situation or problem? Ask yourself: What way could I look at this that would enable me to feel better, more positive, and see a light at the end of the tunnel? Maybe reassuring yourself that there is a solution to your problem, there is help to be found and there is a way forward. This may provide the comfort you need. Another useful phrase to remember is – <u>The perfect way to deal with this person / situation is coming</u>

<u>to me now.</u> And be open and receptive to your inspirational inner guidance. This guidance may come in the form of a thought, an idea, a feeling or a mental picture.

It is amazing how we can keep off that depressing roller-coaster simply by asking ourselves a few questions such as – What feeling is this? What is the healthy solution to this problem? What would I like to do now? And pay attention to the healthy answers. Perhaps these are the questions our well-meaning caregivers did not realise it was important to ask us a long time ago. Ceasing to blame our caregivers for their errors, we as adults are now ready to gladly take responsibility for asking ourselves these 'new' questions that help us heal our emotions and follow our bliss.

The answers to these questions are fundamental to us leading a non-addicted life. Remember to ask yourself – Am I physically hungry? Am I physically full? What feeling am I experiencing now? What words would best describe how I feel right now? And – Given the fact I feel this way what would I like to do now?

It is often enough just to relax physically and acknowledge the feeling, thus confirming the fact that we have no intention of running away from it. You can physically relax even while being active, although if at all possible it is good to sit down in a comfortable chair and ask ourselves those appropriate and meaningful questions, throughout the day as feelings and issues around food and life arise. Thereby helping us analyse and get to the root of the problem more easily. You may very rightly say

– But I do not have the time for such nonsense, I have so many things to do. It is just not possible with my job. When thoughts like this strike, know that an awareness of how you feel is enough, and you can, with patience do that practice of asking yourself these important questions, anywhere. As we become more aware of our feelings, we become expert in feeling comfortable with all our feelings and resolving them with minimum of fuss. To be able to do this, is tremendously freeing and it is a great relief, to be able to go about our day to day life, without being hindered or blocked by emotional garbage. So, let's get busy clearing out and incinerating that metaphorical garbage!

**What would I like to do now?**
This really boils down to good old-fashioned dream chasing! It is okay to chase your dream. In fact you are giving yourself a good chance of catching it! You may say – But is it practical? Will chasing my dream enable me to pay the bills and feed the baby? This is an important question. So let us explore this concept to see if it is valid and worthwhile.
Following your dream is a romantic notion, and many a wonderful film has been based on this concept. In religious terms it means joyously following the guidance of the Holy Spirit, that inner part of us that is linked to God or Source. Certainly a worthy pursuit but again how practical is it for us every day folk, in this material world and money age? Doing what we want, feel inspired to do, like and love has a certain self-

indulgent, almost frivolous connotation. Sometimes children are not allowed to do what they want, even though it may be very creative and constructive. Or maybe as a child you were made to feel guilty about doing what you wanted and sometimes even given the idea that what you wanted was not important compared with the needs of the adults around you.

We, as adults may still feel guilty or even scared about doing what we want and love, having had little experience of doing what we wanted or loved to do as children. This is nothing more than old negative programming which can be changed with the help of positive, consistent and persistent affirmation.

There are some inaccurate associations going around about allowing yourself to do what you want to do. Such as – Well I do not want to go to work, so are you saying that I should not go? - Of course not! What I am saying is – acknowledge your lack of interest in going to work and address that issue. Be aware of what you want from work and from life. You want your work to be something you love and something that is financially rewarding. If a change is required, take the healthy risks needed to bring you good results. Some training in a field you are genuinely interested in perhaps. Ask yourself – Do I want to work in an entirely different field or do I want to work less hours? Can I arrange some evening classes in an activity I enjoy? Would I like to do some evening classes to acquire further education? Do I quite like my work but maybe I would like to plan for a career change in a few years, and what would that require? Is there a personality in my workplace, which I do not like? Would I like to be my own boss?

Asking yourself these probing questions and paying attention to the answers will give you insights, pointers and stirred up enthusiasm, as well as some fears and doubts. The next step, is of course, the mulling over and sorting through of all this. Your inner guidance will help you decide what ideas to act on.

There is also the idea that if we go around doing what we want to do all the time that we would be inconsiderate to the feelings of others, and people will get hurt. One sure way to find out is to ask yourself the obvious question – What do I want from this situation? And – Is this action going to hurt anyone?

When we ask this question, we must be aware if anyone is trying to influence or control us through their actions and reactions. Is a relative or spouse, using their anger to try and control your behaviour, and get you to do what they want?

Stay aware of your own heart-felt desires and feelings, whilst checking in with those nearest and dearest to you, for any ruffled feathers or insecurities. You can reassure your friends and family, if you like, letting them know you are going through changes. Ask for their support and understanding. Thus allowing relationships become more intimate.

So, what we are doing, is giving ourselves permission to be the person we want to be, whilst not allowing other people control us because our actions may go against what they think is best for us. We can still do what we know is in our own best interests to do. It is okay to make positive and healthy changes in our lives, even if someone around us may act hurt or react negatively. Such tactics may be control tactics, born out of their own unresolved emotional issues and fear. Our success may highlight their own unfulfilled dreams. Thus, doing what we want to do, following our dream, taking healthy risks, maybe making a career change could hurt a loved one's ego rather than their true self.

Everyone's true self wants everyone else to be free, to excel and be who they were meant to be. To make their own choices in life and the freedom to make their own mistakes if necessary. Do what you love. Do what you feel is appropriate for you. Do what your positive, creative feelings tell you to do, when those feelings are in accordance with your own personal value system and healthy heartfelt desires.

**For example:** You may feel like sleeping with a certain married man because you are attracted to him, but your personal value system does not agree with that course of action. So, you acknowledge both your feelings and your personal value system but ultimately decide to follow your values because you truly want someone who is available.

Never do what someone else wants you to do, if it goes against your gut instincts. If you do what someone else wants you to do, rather than what you want to do, it will not make either of you happy and you risk greatly damaging yourself and the relationship. Instead, check in with your feelings, acknowledge them, be aware of your personal value system in that area and act wisely and lovingly with strength in your feelings, gut-instincts and personal values. Remember, someone who doesn't hear you say – No – is trying to control you.

This also can be a good time to look at your deep-seated desires and start working your way toward them. Construct a plan of action around them and get busy taking positive steps towards fulfilling that plan. Be flexible. Be present. Be persistent. Be true to yourself.

When we do what we love, we are not only expressing our love and respect for ourselves and those around us, we are also expressing our natural talents and creativity, and that is positively healthy! A far cry from addictive behaviour.

We are in the constant process of assessing and reassessing our values, in each area of our lives. We are now following our dream. We are happily acknowledging and fulfilling our own needs. As we heal, we in fact, become more compassionate towards the struggles of all humankind. We see the needs of others and are in a much better position to encourage, support and constructively empower others to find and take their own steps toward a more fulfilling, creative and joyous life. Long gone are the days of dieting and binge eating. No more controlling others or allowing ourselves to be controlled by others. I say – Hallelujah and Amen to that!

## Tools of Empowerment

The power to move forward, heal and be happy is released through the incorporation into your day to day life, the tools that enable you to feel your feelings rather than suppress them by eating when physically full.

Feelings are neither good nor bad. Even the so called negative feelings such as anger, fear and hate are in themselves not bad. It is not bad to feel these feelings. Uncomfortable – yes, bad – no. These feelings are simply natural. If someone mistreats you over several years, it is not bad to feel hate. We may judge it as bad. We may deny its existence. But if we glimpse a feeling within ourselves it's best to acknowledge it without judgement and most importantly feel it. Above all never say – I shouldn't feel this way. Instead think – Ah, so this is how I feel about so-and-so and this situation. Always validate, seek to understand and heal your own feelings. Thus you validate, seek to understand and heal yourself.

Feelings are energy. And energy can be blocked or free-flowing. The only thing that can be labelled bad, if you like, in that it does indeed bring about some bad results in our lives - is a feeling that is blocked or suppressed. (Suppressed through eating when full). We hold that blocked feeling, in the very cells of our bodies and like water that ceases to flow, it becomes stagnant and a problem. Suppressed feelings are blocked energy. Your blocked energy causes the blocks to your happiness, peace of mind, good health, slimness and fulfilment. The solution is to allow all of your feelings to flow by experiencing them, knowing they do indeed pass and thus dissolving your blocks. Therefore, flowing energy entails you acknowledging your feelings, and taking them into consideration before you take action. Flowing energy is healthy energy. It gives you energy. It educates you and guides you. Like an ever changing symphony, feelings are an intricate part of being human. They are the interface between you and 'out there' life! They literally connect you to life in their invisible but undeniable, very real, way. To dismiss them or wish they were not there just because they are often painful, or uncomfortable, or too intense is foolish. You would be living a half-life if you did not have them, you would be a robot. The value of feelings is immense.

To flow with the emotional symphony of life, learning better and better ways of handling your feelings, is to be guided back to Self – your true self. Feel your feelings, allow their energy to flow through you. This is truly the secret to a happy, healthy, authentic life. In the following pages we will be looking at individual feelings, considering the tools and processes, which enable us to flow with and integrate those feelings most easily. By practicing the suggested tools we empower ourselves to be more at peace with our feelings, and less likely to stuff those feelings down with food eaten when full, or in any other way suppress them. The craving to eat when full is diminished, and our tendency towards addiction dissolves in the light of integrated feelings and cleared energy.

Our ability to be healthy, enjoy life and deal positively with challenges, depends on how we deal with our feelings. It is not so much, what has happened to us in the past, as how we deal with what happened to us in the past. Not so much, the present difficulties themselves, as how we _deal_ with those difficulties.

Not so much the feelings but how we <u>react</u> to those inner feelings, and how we <u>process</u> them. This involves a slight change in focus – We change from focusing on the problem, to focusing on the solution. Negative to positive!

To be able, to deal with whatever life throws our way, without suppressing the feelings associated with it, is our goal. To be able to feel, flow with and integrate our feelings about what life throws at us, is healthier than suppressing these feelings, because in order to suppress the feelings, we have got to do something and that something is - addiction.

It requires a lot of energy to push a feeling into suppression, therefore addiction depletes our energy. Energy, which is ours to use in more positive and enjoyable ways, as we allow ourselves to truly acknowledge our feelings.

**Integration is the opposite of suppression**. Experiencing feelings, even if it feels a bit strange at first, is, I assure you, a most rewarding pursuit, simply because when we are busy experiencing our feelings, we are no longer suppressing them. As we are no longer suppressing them, we are no longer depleting our energy through addiction. If we are not suppressing our feelings, we are not addicts. If we are not eating when physically full then we are not food addicts.

The following tools, not only help us to experience our feelings more comfortably, they also actively encourage and allow the integration of those feelings. Thus we are free to continue daily life, feeling clear, energised and unhindered by uncomfortable feelings and unresolved emotional issues. In relation to food, this is very important. Having learned the alternative to eating when full we no longer turn to food when full in order to suppress what we have learned to deal with in more positive and appropriate ways.

So, let's move forward and take a look at the tools that can help us deal effectively with our feelings and unresolved emotional issues.

## A Tool Kit for Personal Growth – Affirmations

Fifteen minutes of affirmations, either written, thought or spoken aloud, daily is a good idea to start off with. Always make the affirmation in the present tense and positive. The idea being that whatever you want to do be or have, affirm that you are already doing it, being it and having it, regardless of your present reality.

The act of repeatedly writing out, thinking or speaking aloud (in private and out of ear shot of anyone who would ridicule you) a positive affirmation is so powerful that it begins to show you how to change your present conditions into what is repeatedly affirmed. A change of focus, it certainly is. A creative change of focus that encourages new ideas and inspiration to flow forth into your mind simply because you are directing your thinking energy towards a new subject. A desirable subject, a solution, an expanded and wonderful new subject to do with where you wish your life to go. It is, in no uncertain terms, focused attention and what you focus on grows. This focused attention through the repeatedly spoken, thought or written affirmation commences a process of inner acceptance of the improvement you desire and goes about dissolving any psychological blocks. Repeated affirmations, dig gently into the subconscious mind discovering any hidden resentments, fears, doubts or previously suppressed angry, painful feelings, so that we can be aware of and resolve these feelings. Thus freeing up their energy and removing these blocks.

We tend to mentally accept what is continually repeated. So by persistently repeating the positive, the previously suppressed negative, thoughts and feelings can be uncovered, released and replaced with the acceptance of that positive truth, repeatedly affirmed. The results of which are no less than increased understanding and satisfaction, feelings of relief and ultimately advancement and enlightenment for the powerful inner work and cleansing that you yourself have done!

## Attitude, Affirmations and Visualisations

It is said that what is repeatedly pictured and spoken aloud can manifest in one's life. Take a few moments now, and consider what you habitually think about, talk about and visualise for yourself. Do you worry rather than having faith and trust in the goodness of life? Do you complain rather than being grateful? Do you dwell on what could go wrong rather than dwell on what could go right? Do you waste time thinking of the lack in your life rather than noticing the abundance, even if it is only an abundance of air to breathe?

May be all you have in abundance along with air, is a large container of salt. It is an abundance of something. What is the use of having salt in abundance you may ask? The point is that most of us can afford this item and owning it, how do you consider yourself? The grateful owner of this abundance of salt, knowing that at least all your salt needs are taken care of for the next six months? Or are you the helpless pauper with salt? More than likely you have much more in your life than that, maybe not. You could be heavily in debt, and in great despair. What I am saying is – The way we view, what life has given us, is where our power lies. You have no doubt heard the phrase: If life gives you lemons then make lemonade! This is a perfect example of the point I wish to make. So, between the salt and the homemade lemonade, we can begin with a grateful heart and work on changing our outer reality, for the better, by thinking abundance, affirming abundance, and visualising abundance, regardless of what lack we may be facing. Through the daily practice of affirmation and visualisation, we have the tools, to take ourselves from limited, depressed thinking and results, to unlimited, uplifted thinking and results. In other words, all of us have the power – through the gifts of daily affirmation and visualisation – to take ourselves from lack to abundance.

So, affirm what you desire. Every day affirm – I am slim – for 5 to 15 mins daily. And visualise your heartfelt desire, visualise yourself slim, visualise the life you would love to lead. Visualise your relationships and career as this slim woman. Visualise the clothes you would wear and how good you would feel. Make it very positive. Remember you can't have too much, for you can always give it away. Visualise in colour and in detail if possible and summon up the good vibes of that ideal life. Take a piece of paper and write down your visualisation, at the bottom of the page write the following affirmation – 'With gratitude and acceptance I move forward in life. This is what I desire. I deserve it and I can have it, regardless of the past. The highest good now becomes a reality for myself and for everyone involved. I am a slim healthy woman.' A simple formula for powerful results!

Our power to overcome unwanted experiences and become a victor, lies in our positive approach. It is not always easy, for obviously ploughing through difficult emotional debris that we would rather not be aware of, or feel, is work – inner work that brings solid and lasting outer results.

From where you are now, develop a positive faith-filled approach. The attitude of positive faith. Faith in the good. Faith in health and healing in all areas of life, is what gets positive results. This is a basic truth, which is essential to a happy life, no matter what you have experienced in the past, or are dealing with in the present; the attitude of positive faith is your tool for success. Have faith that you have the courage and the right to make the choices that are in tune with your own heart-felt desires, regardless of what others think you should be doing. Have faith in the highest good manifesting for everyone involved. Hold on to this precious truth. It can see you through to your own personal victories!

Feelings derive from our thoughts and both our conscious and subconscious belief systems. Put simply, if we think unhappy thoughts, we feel unhappy, whereas if we think happy thoughts we feel happy. Repeatedly thinking happy thoughts and speaking happy words in the form of affirmations, results in a basically happy belief system, which in turn results in happy, joyous feelings and occurrences in one's life.

'This all sounds too simple and basic!' – You may exclaim. Basic and simple it is. Effective and practical to the person who dares to apply such simple ideas into his or her own life and demand the positive results they so rightly deserve!

Notice how many of the following thoughts you habitually think or would consider being your basic belief system:

No matter what happens I know I can handle it and learn from the experience.

Wonderful things happen to me!

I acknowledge everything just as it is and I can change what I want to change.

I am glad to be alive and I transcend the problems that life gives me.

I am doing it right, I am supported, I am rewarded. I want to be here.

I am strong, I am healthy, I am prosperous and I am grateful.

Life is good. Life is sweet. People are basically good. However I can deal with troublesome people and situations with ease and grace. I love life.

I love and appreciate myself for who I am right now.

Peace, love, wisdom and perfect solutions come to me, through my connection to Spirit. I am peaceful. I am joyous.

That was an example of a very healthy, joyous, positive belief system. The more joyous and positive the thoughts you constantly hold in your mind, the more joyous and positive you feel. What goes around comes around. Since what you send out is what comes back to you multiplied, the results of your sending out all those positive feelings will be very rewarding in terms of happy, positive experiences in life.

If you are aware that you may have negative thoughts and beliefs systems, and would like to hold more positive ones, all you need do is use the tools of affirmations coupled with visualisation to notice the positive results.

Say 'No' to your excess weight. Say 'No' to your eating disorder. Every time you eat when you are not physically hungry, you are saying 'Yes' to having an eating disorder. Begin to say 'No' to having an eating disorder by affirming the following – 'I no longer fear getting fat. I now heal this eating disorder and addiction to food when full. I deserve to lose weight and be slim. I now pinpoint and resolve the emotional issues that cause me to eat when full. I now lose excess weight permanently and naturally. I am patient. I understand why I would eat when full and I now stop when full 100% of the time. I am slim.'

Affirm: I (…your name…) can lose weight and heal this eating disorder. It is safe for me to lose weight and be slim. I say 'No' to a life of excess weight and compulsive eating. I am now willing to feel my feelings, and resolve my emotional issues. I am now willing to be slim. I now uncover and heal any subconscious worries or concern I may have about becoming the slim, attractive woman. I now dissolve any blocks to my attaining and maintaining my own perfectly, slim, natural weight.

You can use these affirmations when you feel doubt, despair or hopelessness about not being able to overcome the eating disorder. The above affirmations will help you develop a healthier and more empowering attitude toward healing this complex problem.

The power of Affirmations - Being aware of and working in the present moment is the way to take back control of your life and improve your future. Writing or declaring affirmations is some of the most effective work you can do in the present moment to change your inner thoughts and belief systems that are not serving you well. Doing this inner work with affirmations has the effect of transforming self-defeating beliefs into life-enhancing beliefs. That is how anyone can create a future where they experience work they love, financial security, nurturing relationships, joy, peace, good health, a slim body and fulfilment.

Do not underestimate the power of persistent and consistent affirmation.

Forgiveness: A New-Age approach and an ancient law! The daily practice of forgiveness enables us to lighten that suppressed emotional load we carry around with us, which inevitably manifests in us as addictions, relationship, health or financial problems.

**Why forgive?**
A forgiveness affirmation is one of the most powerful affirmations you can make. It is an inner cleanser, clearing out the bitterness, pain, sorrow and resentments of the past; and let's face it, we all have some of that! Declaring forgiveness for yourself and those who have hurt you, or those with whom you are angry, is the most effective healing technique available today – and it is free! Forgiveness gives you the power of peace. It gives you the alternative to retaliation. On a personal level, you can avoid a negative reaction to a hurtful situation, no arguments, no domestic disputes. On a world-wide level, no retaliation, no wars, instead the quiet calm of peaceful resolving.

Question: Will this forgiveness business not make me a victim? Answer: Consider if you will, this universal truth – What you send out comes back to you multiplied. Send out forgiveness and love – forgiveness and love come back to you multiplied. Not necessarily from the same people, in fact, more than likely you will be distancing yourself from some of those you are forgiving. The love, friendship and peace will come from new friends and situations.

For example: You slap me in the face. I have two choices. I can feel angry and slap you back either physically or verbally, or I can feel angry but walk away and forgive you, resolving to avoid you in the future!

Considering what we send out comes back to us multiplied, I acknowledge my feelings, feel my feelings, maybe even tell you my feelings, and explain that I will not tolerate such treatment, but I also forgive you knowing that forgiveness comes back to me multiplied. Your slap comes back to you multiplied. The universe will slap you back, maybe not literally but in the most appropriate way, in the fulfilment of the universal law, what you send out comes back to you multiplied. It might be quite useful to remember this if ever you feel like retaliating . No matter what has happened to us in the past, continued abuse is not the answer that anyone is seeking. Forgiveness is!

Some of my clients have asked me if forgiveness does not mean that we are suppressing our feelings. To ensure further suppression of your feelings does not happen, all that is necessary, is an awareness of your feelings before and as you are repeating the forgiveness affirmations. Be willing to stay focused on your feelings and you can be sure that you are not suppressing them. Forgiveness, is in fact a tool, which can both, put us in touch with previously suppressed, angry, resentful or painful feelings and help us resolve those feelings.

One of my clients tried forgiving some people and found the feelings of relief and resolve. Surprised at the quick and positive results asked me how forgiveness does this resolving so effectively. I had to admit, this is one question I cannot answer, except to say that it is the mystery of forgiveness. It is a law of the universe and it works.

When we ask: 'Does this person deserve my forgiveness?' We are focusing inappropriately. Instead focus on the answer to this question: 'Do I deserve the benefits that forgiving others can give me?' – Yes!

If you have never tried forgiveness affirmations then you obviously have not experienced their vast benefits first hand. Maybe you have read books recommending forgiveness as a tool for personal growth, or know of someone who has had good results from practicing the forgiveness technique. Either way, the best way to find out about the benefits of practicing daily forgiveness in terms of increased wellbeing, is to try it for yourself.

There is nothing like first-hand experience to prove, to yourself, what works best for you! It is said that the person who does not forgive burns a bridge over which he himself must cross one day. Not a wise thing to do!

Look at it this way – when you do not forgive the person with whom you are angry, you bind yourself to that person with hoops of steel. Forgiveness is the only thing strong enough to dissolve those hoops of steel, leaving you free from that person forever. Now that is a good idea!

So, I ask you: Do you deserve the benefits forgiveness offers? I think you do.

## Why should I make the time to forgive others?

Do you want to be bound with hoops of steel to a person you dislike or hate? I think not! Then forgiveness is our metaphysical and practical answer. Persistent forgiveness allows you to become the person to whom the mistakes of the past have no detrimental effect. It is like it never happened.

A few things to remember about forgiveness:
1. It does **not** mean you condone the act you are forgiving.
2. It is claiming a divorce from past unhappiness.
3. It heals bitterness, pain, anger, unhappiness, resentment, fear, grief and hate.
4. It is the means by which we can break negative cycles of behaviour.
5. It is an inner cleanser, cleansing us of any difficult emotions.
6. It allows you to feel better, more so than the one you are forgiving.
7. The one you are forgiving may pick up on it subconsciously, and as a result, react to you in more positive ways.
8. When we forgive someone, our relationship with him or her either gets better or ends. You gain the emotional power to do what it takes to leave that person or situation.

9. Forgiveness affirmations, written or spoken aloud when you are alone, means you do not have to speak to the one you are forgiving. You may never want to see them again, that is okay. It is best that you have only loving, trustworthy people around you.

10. Forgiveness affirmations help you process your feelings about the way they treated you. Forgiveness allows you to learn an important lesson and be stronger.

11. Forgiveness forms a metaphysical vacuum. Nature abhors a vacuum. Your desired good rushes in to fill that vacuum.

**Anger:** How to tap into your anger power and turn it into purposefulness. Anger, like all emotions, in itself is not negative. It is how we deal with our anger that either helps or hinders our personal growth. Anger, is an automatic and natural reaction to situations, which are unfair, cruel, abusive or harmful. Anger carriers the message – something is not quite right here. We usually feel angry when our needs are not being met appropriately. When we listen to, acknowledge and act on our anger appropriately, we are guided to happiness. The following tools are suggested ways of enabling us to feel, experience and integrate our anger effectively, so that it actually empowers us.

It is particularly useful to be aware of your own anger, because once you allow yourself to feel your anger and integrate it, it becomes purposefulness. Remember feeling a feeling automatically allows that feeling to integrate. Flowing feelings allow integration of feelings. Integration is the opposite of suppression. Integrating our feelings is our healthy alternative to the binge which suppresses our feelings.

Anytime you find yourself angry, ask yourself some or all of the following questions. This will help you look at your anger, understand it and integrate it more easily. Thus allowing your energy to flow and become the positive, powerful force in your life, actively helping you to accomplish your goals.

You can ask yourself these questions whilst looking back on past angry experiences or to help you deal with present ones:
What did I want from this situation?
What specifically, about this situation made me angry?
What did I expect to happen in this situation?
Would walking away from this situation have helped me?
Was I expecting someone to act differently?
Was how they actually acted similar to how one of my parents acts?
Was I giving them my power? Were they trying to make me do something I did not want to do?
If so how could I have acted differently in order to stay empowered and get the result I wanted?
Does something about this situation remind me of how I was treated as a child?
Was I fearful, under all that anger?
Was I sad or grief stricken too?

In other words if I had left the situation and just felt my anger instead of expressing it, would the angry feelings have given way to fearful or sad feelings?

Was there something I was fearful of doing or saying?

What was I afraid would happen?

Was I expecting the other person to do something that I am not doing for myself?

Were my feelings and needs being acknowledged by the other person in that situation?

Did I acknowledge my own needs in that situation?

What did I do to get my needs fulfilled?

Were my needs being met in that situation?

What was the issue? Protection, respect, responsibility, being listened to or accepted?

Was this also and issue for me when I was growing up?

Was I around other people who were suppressing their feelings, maybe their anger or fear and I was picking up that suppressed energy?

Suppression of anger results in depleted purposefulness. People who suppress their anger often lack purposefulness. Maybe they wish to accomplish a certain goal or dream or simply have a nicer life, but they never manage to achieve it. It is difficult to fulfil your dreams when you lack purposefulness. When you suppress your anger you are robbing yourself of your own purposefulness.

The valuable message of that anger is - something is wrong and you need to be purposeful to correct that wrong.

Through experiencing your own anger, and learning how to deal with it healthily, you regain your purposefulness.

When angry with someone: Step back, acknowledge your anger and use one of the following.

Call – 'Time out!' Tell the other person there is something you have to sort out for yourself and that you are taking a 'time out' to think.

Walk out of the room. Walk around the block. Give yourself a couple of hours or a couple of days. Even have a vacation or weekend away. Ask yourself: What do I want from this situation? Allow yourself to acknowledge how you feel.

Remember God, Goddess, Allah, Buddha, Jesus, Angels or Saints (what or whomever you believe in as a higher benevolent power) and call on them silently for help. No matter how angry you are feeling remembering your own spirituality, and reaffirming your connection with that higher power, helps keep you centred so that you can rise above the problem and find the perfect solution.

Distance yourself from the person who is making you angry and beat the mattress or sofa when you are alone. Then write down what you want. This helps clarify things for you.

Leave the room stating that you are going to seek legal advice / professional advice / a second opinion.

Give your anger the blessing of forgiveness.

The daily practice of forgiveness is both empowering and practical. A valuable tool for a busy technological and spiritual age. It is for people of all walks of life. Anyone can do it, fat or slim, rich or poor. Prince or pauper! The daily practice of forgiveness allows us to dig into out subconscious mind, find any previously hidden, blocked feelings and let them go, once and for all.

Forgiveness gets us to the safe and wonderful place, where all the negative experiences of past and present have no ill effects. The good has been born from past and present traumas and anger. Through forgiveness affirmations, we let the relief of burdens be our goal. You can be strong, well-loved and nurtured regardless of the past. The habit of forgiveness grows easily, and gives you the power to be free from your past and joyously create a new way of life full of positive experiences.

**Tools that help us deal with our anger healthily**

When you get angry, instead of stuffing it down with food when full, use one of these useful alternatives to help you deal with your anger in a healthy way:

1. Forgive whomever you are angry with. Repeat a forgiveness affirmation verbally, or written, until you experience a sense of relief.

2. Do 'The Work' of Byron Katie. She has a free worksheet from her website - thework.com - and you can research her method on You Tube.

3. Before sleep spend half an hour doing a mental review of your day and forgive anyone with whom you are out of harmony. This is the way to clear out, not only anger but also bitterness, suppressed unhappiness, pain, hostility, resentment,

hate or frustration. If you feel someone has treated you unfairly forgive him or her. If someone has hurt you physically or emotionally distance yourself from them.

4. Do the forgiveness prayers of Howard Wills – Free from his website: Howardwills.com

5. Do the Ho'oponopono Mantra – it is on You Tube

All these methods help you process your feelings – feelings you may have previously stuffed down with food when full. They help you change suppressed feelings, which you carry around all day, into flowing, energising, feelings which enable you to function effectively, gain added insight into people, their actions and yourself. Thus allowing you to be more emotionally present in life, learn from life and gain gems of wisdom and love from every aspect of your life.

6. If you are angry with yourself, forgive yourself. Self-forgiveness is equally important to forgiving others. Know you did the best you could and be willing to do it differently next time. You'll be able to do it differently because you are a different person now through self-awareness and self-forgiveness.

7. Relax physically. Visualise yourself like a jellyfish completely floppy and loose. Allow every muscle in your body to relax. It is very hard to shout at someone when relaxed. In the heat of the moment, if you realise that you are being triggered and become aware that staying calm and/or walking away will be a better move than yelling, and you'll have come a

long way. Being physically relaxed helps you be calm enough to stay in control and walk away without negating your feelings. You are also more likely to find a realistic solution to the problem at hand, because when you are physically relaxed you can be more aware of the precious guidance coming from your intuition.

8. If you find yourself angry because of a situation affirm – 'I have faith that divine love is alive and working in this situation now, resolving it, healing it and blessing all concerned. Light, love and wisdom now provide the solution. I see the perfect solution clearly now.' Only through use can you feel and experience the positive force of a repeated faith affirmation.

The above affirmation works equally well for anger that is felt towards a loved one who has not behaved or responded to you in the way you would have liked them to. You can repeat a forgiveness affirmation to yourself, there and then, or wait until later when, in private, you can affirm aloud.

9. Ask yourself: 'Is this situation, event, or feeling reminding me of some past painful memory?' If so, some forgiveness affirmations for those involved in that earlier memory, can help you release that painful memory and process it's associated feelings. (Again please remember, you do not have to say directly to that person that you are forgiving them. They would only laugh or ridicule you. This is private work you do on your own to cleanse out the toxicity of the interaction from within you and help you gain some clarity and strength.) Thus you peel back and heal layer upon layer of previously wounded consciousness. You

become aware of, and resolve the root cause of your own painful feelings. Through forgiving the original root transgressor you also dissolve the root of your present day problem, miraculously clearing it up for good.

Ask yourself: Is someone treating me with disrespect? Am I treating myself with a lack of respect?' Remember people around us are our mirrors. Especially our loved ones.

We all subconsciously pick up on any suppressed feelings coming from our partner or friends and will often subconsciously act out that feeling in our subconscious efforts to help them resolve these feelings and emotional issues. Knowing this is very important.

Example: If you partner gets angry with you regularly then it is worth thinking about this a little more deeply. Is he mirroring your own suppressed anger? How will you know? Well firstly, open up a dialogue with your inner child. Is she angry? This is very healing and enlightening and can clear up a lot of previously suppressed feelings very effectively, also allowing your intimate relationship develop easily or end easily enough.

It is also worth acknowledging that it is abusive to habitually yell and scream at someone, slam your hands down on the table or desk, to give them 'the look' or the silent treatment, all abusive offshoots of anger and control tactics to boot! If you or your partner are doing this, you are in trouble and it would be a good idea to read 'Men Who Hate Women and the Women Who Love

Them' by Susan Harris. It is an informative and interesting book on the behaviour of angry controlling men and their partners. The book offers real insights and practical tools for combating this behaviour.

Ask yourself: What am I expecting this person to do that I am not doing for myself? Then get busy doing it!

10.     Beat your mattress. Beat pillows! Buy yourself several big cushions or pillows and beat them with your fists. You can even buy a punch bag! A great way to harmlessly and quickly vent your anger when no one is around. Thus letting it go, and wallow in the relief of having healthily processed your anger.

**Recommended reading for dealing with anger**
The Dance of Anger by Harriet Goulder-Learner
Families and How to Survive Them by Robin Skinner and John Cleese
The Dynamic Laws of Healing by Catherine Ponder
Venus and Mars Starting Over by John Gray
Audio: Releasing Anger by Louise Hay

I realise that joy gives me the power to correct my mistakes. Joy and trust and courage are linked. Joy can be experienced as a spiritual foundation based on knowledge of spiritual truths. The truth of an abundant, supportive universe. The truth of the innate power within each of us that is divine in nature, otherwise known as the Spirit of Joy. Lack of recognition of this inner divine joy (even if it is only a tiny spark) can lead to a multitude of ills.

Joy is no flamboyant, frivolous creature. It is a magnificent quality born of light and beyond circumstance. Joy exists beyond appearances of lack and even hardship. It exists within these experiences because it exists within you. Joy is born of forgiveness, love, praise and gratitude. Joy is brought to the fore by doing what you love and standing up for your own personal goals and dreams. Joy is the essential ingredient in the celebration cake of life. You may say – Well I don't want a flat pancake for a life! So how do I get that celebration cake instead?

It is said that in order to have joy we must be able to experience the full extent of our suffering; and I believe this is a key to overcoming depression. Feeling our suffering allows it to integrate. Feeling our suffering allows it to pass. The help of a therapist is often good in working through particularly difficult things that have caused you suffering. I personally found Rebirthing Breathwork and the Breathing Techniques of Wim Hoff to be excellent.

Anger too, is very much linked with depression. In fact depression is often the result of suppressed anger. Therefore, in order to overcome depression one must deal with one's anger. Binge eating may be your means of suppressing your anger. So reading again the previous pages for further insight remembering depression can be a symptom of suppressed anger. Deal with your suppressed anger and you heal your depression.

Affirm – No, I do not accept any illness as part of my present or future life. Nothing but healing comes into my life right now. I have faith in my own healing. Healing light is within me and around me now.

Chris Griscom, author, global spiritual leader, visionary and founder of The light Institute in Galisteo, New Mexico also talks of asking the body what colour it needs, as each colour has a healing frequency, and you simply visualise that colour flooding your body and notice how you feel.

## Make time to make merry

Making merry is not just for Christmas, and finding fun is such a simple technique to enable us to keep depression at bay that it is sometimes overlooked or dismissed as trivial. As we focus on the lighter side of life, on those little joys such as reading the funnies in a newspaper and watching sit-coms or comedy films, it goes a long way to lift the spirits, calm the mind and let a healing balm flow through the cells of the body. The practice of praising also raises the spirits when practiced daily. Mentally praise yourself for getting up in the morning. Quietly praise your kitchen, your cabinets with food, your running water and electric light without griping about the bills. Counting your blessings if you like, notice the everyday miracles all around. Let life's problems melt into the distance as a change of perspective has worked it's magic.

We can put ourselves in a more open and receptive frame of mind to find solutions to our problems. We all have problems, but we sometimes forget, to our detriment, that we all have <u>solutions</u> too. So now we are just learning how to find them, and in so doing, whatever we are experiencing seems manageable, we gain the opportunity to see the big picture and even have some intuitive guidance about what to do next. Through following that intuition, and overcoming the problem, strength is gained. We are blessed with a glimpse of the lesson we learned in our time of trial. Our sense of security increases in knowing that we can 'go through' whatever life gives us no matter how unpleasant or unwanted that experience. We go through our pain, sorrow, anger, depression and fear to a place of higher energy, more love and increased wisdom. It gives us confidence and strength when we go through and discover the joys of life. We may have to look hard for them. We often need to persist in looking for the good, but still seek! Seek joy, pleasantness and beauty for through focusing on these, lies the cure, for a multitude of life's ills both big and small.

Two things to remember about happiness

1. Happiness is not a luxury. It is a necessity!
2. Happiness is the result of doing what you love. It is also the result of being self-determined. In other words – you making decisions and taking action that is in line with your own desires, intuition, beliefs, ethics, wants and needs.

I truly believe that depression is strongly linked to not doing what you truly desire to do and not following your own personal value system. Decide where you stand, what you will and will not tolerate in terms of family, career, love and leisure. Think about your values and standards in each of these areas. Write down what you desire and what your priorities are in each of these areas. Create your own value system. When you know what is right and appropriate for yourself, you have your own value system. When we make decisions for ourselves, based on our own value system and we ensure, that what we do is in line with those values, then we get to feel connected and empowered in our environment. We get to feel real. If we simply do what another person tells us to do, when it is not in line with our own personal values, then we get to feel powerless. We feel a lack of validity and connection within our own environment. Any normal person feels anger about being powerless and if these feelings are suppressed by eating when full then the result is depression. Consciously healing your wounds, establishing your own value system and acting in line with it, automatically leads to fulfilment and a sense of authenticity about what you do. Now that is rewarding and what self-determination is all about.

**Recommended reading for overcoming depression**
The Dynamic Laws of Healing Catherine Ponder
Feeling Good – New Mood Therapy. The clinically proven drug-free treatment for depression by David D Burns Published by 'Avon'

## Boredom

All our boredom is trying to tell us is that we would like to be doing something else. In other words boredom's message is – I'd like to do something different to what I am doing right now. I'd like to be doing something more in harmony with my own likes and interests. But our fears get in the way. Doing something new, like attending an evening class is part and parcel of allowing 'new' habits come into our lives and replace old dysfunctional ones. Doing something new instead of eating when physically full, usually involves feeling a little scared.

Fear of just going forth, changing and advancing, often stems from childhood experience. We picked up our parents fears and maybe were even held back from venturing forth into the new. Know that it is not okay to hold yourself back when you are in you thirties (for example) and wish to join an evening class in a subject you like, or spend a little time in the pool, or go for a walk every morning or start to write a journal or a book, waking up an hour earlier to do so.

Boredom tells us to take action and be sensitive to our environment and the wonder of even the smallest of things that give you pleasure. Increasing conscious awareness by practicing living in the 'now' and moving from your head to your heart, from thinking to feeling. Following up on involving yourself in what you love to do, persisting in doing what you are interested in, kills boredom, for your life becomes magical. You take courage and maybe even be surprised at how much courage it takes to join a simple pottery class but don't let that dissuade

you. The fear goes as soon as you start, and gives way to the new world you've entered - a world filled with what interests you!
There is layer upon layer of feelings and emotional issues to be felt and navigated if you like, in this experience of living. But that is what giving up eating when physically full is all about, learning to trust your navigational skills, while exploring unknown waters, until you find that paradise island.

## Doubts and fear

I read somewhere that one who conquers doubt and fear also conquers failure. So how to handle fear? Well this is not a matter of getting rid of feelings or suddenly having things easy. Life is about having emotions and feelings. Truly living is about having and solving problems, or as I like to call them – challenges. If we would like to make life in any sense easier, then what we can do, is work with the challenges, rather than resisting, resenting or running away from them, as we tend to do when we eat compulsively or in any other way suppress our feelings. I have mentioned before and it is worth repeating – the main key to achieving a more satisfactory or easier life, lies in how we deal with our feelings, emotional issues and challenges.

Fear is an important one, for this feeling alone can sometimes prevent us from moving logically and healthily forward in career, relationships, personal growth and health. Also, when we integrate our fear, we get enthusiastic preparation for the future. In other words, once related to appropriately, our fear can actually help us move forward in life. The important thing is to feel it! Feel the fear and remember fear is the absence of love. Then take these simple steps to deal appropriately with this powerful feeling.

## Ten tools for dealing with fear

1.	Faith. Faith in love and goodness overcomes fear. Positive faith-filled thoughts and wise loving thoughts all have the power to conquer fear. They give you the power to move if you need to move, or stay if you need to stay. They give you the power to make wise decisions and be safe.

2.	Analyse the fear. We can conquer fear through knowledge, so do analyse your fear. Ask yourself – 'Is this fear rational or irrational?' If it is irrational ask yourself – 'Where did this feeling come from? Is it to do with my past? Could something frightening have happened to me, in the past, in a similar situation? Am I being triggered?'

3.	If the fear is rational then take appropriate steps to address this fear. Is it, for example – a fear of being burgled, when your house has poor security? Then appropriately addressing this fear might involve thinking about installing an alarm or joining a neighbourhood watch scheme.

4.	Ask yourself – 'What would I say to comfort a small frightened child?' – Say this to yourself.

5.	Affirm this to overcome any fear you have around your eating disorder – 'I am willing to release my fears of becoming slim. I am willing to release my fears of becoming fat. I have faith that I now have the power to heal this eating disorder, lose excess weight easily, permanently, healthily and naturally. I have faith that my slim self is now emerging safely and in peace. I am healed. I am slim.

6. When fear or doubt strikes say to yourself – 'What would be a reassuring thought with which to address this fear or doubt? You have got yourself another helpful affirmation.

7. Sometimes we experience fear from the past. If we were separated from our mother at birth or during the following days, as was common (and highly inappropriate) hospital policy – it was traumatic for the new born 'you'. You could have suppressed fear around that forgotten event. This is what is known a birth trauma and we all, to a greater or lesser extent, have some. Again rebirthing breathwork is the effective solution here. Forgiveness affirmations for the doctor or midwives also help you clear up that trauma and, believe it or not, can help heal issues with authority figures because that doctor and midwife were you first encounter with authority. If it was traumatic it lays a blueprint for fear of authority.

8. If there was a lot of fearful emotions around when you were a child, such as fear of whether there was enough money for food and bills. Fear of a parent losing a job or being unable to find and keep one. Then fear could be somewhat of a normal feeling for you. Fear could have been around, when you were a child regardless of whether your parents were rich or poor. Financial wealth is no guarantee of lack of fear about always being abundantly supplied. The trick, to help deal with this type

of fear, is to develop a confidence in your ability to handle whatever life gives you, be it poverty or wealth. The truth is you can deal with whatever comes along. Actually believing that, enables it to become an evident reality in your life.

When you pinpoint a specific fear thought such as – There isn't enough money – turn it into a positive opposite and affirm – There is always enough money – until you believe it and see it as a reality in your life.

9.   Bible quotes are particularly powerful to affirm or meditate on when one is fearful. This one is a favourite of mine 'There shall no evil befall thee, neither shall any plague come nigh thy tent, for He will give His Angels charge over thee to keep thee in all thy ways.' (Psalms 91:10, 11).

Through verbally or mentally repeating a quote such as this you are conjuring up the feeling of safety and protection as well as the calm ability to do all you need to do to keep safe. A sure antidote for a fearful frame of mind.

10.   Your fears could come from some unconscious fearful thought patterns about life, or unconscious conclusions you made in childhood. Again I suggest rebirthing breathwork as the most effective ways to uncover and help resolve these particularly difficult feelings and subconscious root causes.

**The 'I have faith' process**
Take a pen a paper and finish these sentences.
List A
In my relationship, I am afraid of …

In my career, I am afraid of…
In my life, I am afraid of…
In my financial affairs, I am afraid of…
As regards my health, I am afraid of…

Now, I would like you to construct a series of sentences with – 'I have faith that…' And fill in the opposite concept to the fear, as in the examples which follow.

In my relationship, I have faith that…
In my career, I have faith that…
In my life, I have faith that…
As regards my health, I have faith that…

**Example:**
In my relationship I am afraid my husband will leave me. Turn your fear into its opposite like this – I have faith that my husband is faithful. I have faith we can handle what life gives us, faithfulness or lack of, being together or amicably splitting.
This way you are not in denial of life's trials and tribulations, but also you are not allowing anything that comes your way (wanted or unwanted) to cause you to eat when full or feel destroyed by it.
**Example:**
In my career, I am afraid that I will not earn enough money, even though I work hard.

Turn this around to… I have faith that I can be abundantly provided for in many ways, even miraculous ways, and I have faith that I have wisdom in earning and spending my money so all my needs are met.

**The 'Something has always stopped me' process**
Ask yourself: What have I always wanted to do? Write down some of the things you have always wanted to do but have never done. In other words list your desires. This is your big dream. Your biggest dream. The dream life, the dream relationship, the dream holiday or the dream career. Whatever your goal may be, no matter how impossible, improbable or down right unrealistic the attainment of it may seem, it does not matter. Think big. Think – What would I do, if there was nothing (and I mean nothing!) to stop you?
Example:
1. Buy a BMW
2. Go to South America for a holiday to see the Mayan Pyramids
3. Become an air hostess
Good now select one of your desires and write it down.
Example: South American holiday to see the Mayan Pyramids.
Then ask yourself: What is the first step towards achieving this goal?
Answer: Saving the money to pay for it.

Now make this your new goal and ask yourself: What three or more steps could help me feel as if I am on my way to accomplishing this goal?

Answer: Opening a separate saving account. Get a part time job / overtime / weekend work to provide me with extra income to save. Have a clear out and sell unwanted items on eBay or at the local Car Boot Sale.

What can I do to prepare myself for the reality of this dream?

I can get some brochures from the local travel agent. I can check out the different deals on the internet. I can buy new luggage. I can decide whether I want to travel alone or with a friend or in a group.

Now write a detailed description of the way you want it to unfold. The perfect holiday with the perfect companions and ease and flow all the way throughout. Including informative guides, friendly staff, great weather and breath-taking scenery.

Visualise this description often.

If fears come up then ask: Well how can I deal with this fear? Maybe the fear is telling you – Don't go alone on this trip, go with a friend or with an organised excursion, it will be safer. Always make a wise choice, take healthy risks, not foolish ones. Be aware, pay attention to what you really want. You may, funnily enough, find out through this inner enquiry that simply a week touring several sacred sites in England is enough to satisfy that particularly dream. We can be flexible in finding our answers.

Remember – experiencing the dark stuff is a necessary part of healing. That dark stuff is what we are running away from and suppressing with food when full. To heal, and live the life of a recovered compulsive eater, we must stop running away. We must stand still, face and feel our fears in order to overcome them effectively. The refreshing truth is – We can all do it, once we face up to fear, it can dissolve.

And finally ask yourself – In what ways do I help myself feel safe?

**For Example:**
I read the 91st Psalm
I reassure myself. Give myself a little pep talk.
If there is a decision to be made, I give myself time to think even if others are pressuring me to take a certain course of action.
I tune into or visualise a spiritual, protecting presence within me or surrounding me.

**Recommended Reading:**
Feel the Fear and Do It Anyway Susan Jeffers
The Course In Miracles
Love is Letting Go of Fear Gerard Jampolski
Why Am I Afraid to Tell You Who I Am? John Powell

**Confusion**
Confusion can arise from not being consciously aware of your wants and needs in the various situations that life throws at you. Confusion also can arise from not knowing what you want from

a person in your life, or not having the courage to ask for what you want from that person. We may feel confused (and guilty) when we do not do what we really want to do. Such as taking an art class, when we really want to study law, just because our parents are in favour of artistic pursuits. Or, when under pressure from midwives allow your baby to be weighed at birth when there is no medical reason to do so, and you really want to wait three or four days before weighing him, as it is perfectly safe to do so and less traumatic for the new-born and you. You do things you do not want to do, and feel confused, upset, unsupported and depressed even. You do things you do not really want to do because you are afraid of what others will think or do, you are afraid of displeasing people. Wondering why people, who are supposed to love and support you, are not loving and supporting you. They are leaving you feeling like your needs are somehow 'wrong' or unimportant and that they know best. This really is a power struggle, and you are dealing with people who have their own agenda, and are manipulative about implementing that agenda. This can be an upsetting and confusing time as you sort out what is best for you and your loved ones. A time to honestly ask yourself - Who is to be trusted and who is to be let go of? This can be painful to discover but necessary in order for the fog to clear and right action in line with your own heart-felt truth to prevail.

Therefore courage – feeling the fear while doing what is in line with your own personal value system is what is required on the journey out of confusion.

Allow yourself to listen to that still small voice within, so you can know what it is that you truly want. Follow up on the ideas you get from that inner knowing. Try different evening classes, travel, follow your instincts, gut feelings and intuitions. Have the courage to go for it and chase your dreams. Now, I did not say it would be easy, some parts of this journey are uphill and difficult. Mistakes can be made. You may have to face your own personal dragons and fears. That is why courage is needed, but the good news is that you do not even need to feel courageous, just start, make a move in the direction of your goal and it will all fall into place as you learn from your mistakes, move forward and grow.

Remember your connection to your inner guidance system becomes stronger as you give up eating when full and follow the 'Am I hungry?' guidelines at the beginning of this book. Memorise a favourite uplifting quote such as - 'Every day in every way things are getting better and better for me now.' Recite it when you feel afraid. Reassure yourself that you can have what you want and desire in life, that you deserve to get your needs met. Know that something greater than you, the people in your life and the situations in your life, can and is supporting you as you learn and grow. Affirm that the highest good is manifesting for all concerned effortlessly. Affirm this Catherine Ponder quote 'Something good shall come from this; things are getting better and better for me now.'

When you start thinking about improving your life, wanting better health, warmer more nurturing relationships, or a new career, do not be surprised if it gets a bit confusing at times. Often we avoid asking ourselves probing questions simply because it is too uncomfortable and it seems like there is too much to sort out. Too many choices. Too many thoughts and feelings of uncertainty. Too many obstacles to even consider moving forward in life. So, if confusion rears its ugly head, at any time, as you are searching within for your future, be assured the simple way through confusion is magically concealed in a pen and notebook!

Yes, getting it down on paper! Your ideas. Your dreams. Your hopes and desires. Your greatest wishes for yourself and others. List your way out of confusion. Avoid thinking or writing out long pages of self-doubt and negativity. Do not limit your dreams. Think unlimited, positive and simple. Write down only what you want to happen. Make one list of what you want in life. Make another list of what you want in your family relationships. Another list of what you want in your friendships. Another list for what you want in your work / career. Another list for romance and yet another list for your health. You get the idea! Have as many lists for as many areas of life that you wish to cover.

Next look at you lists at least once a week. If you want to change, re-arrange, add to, or delete anything on any one of your lists do so. Have fun with this. Allow planning your future to excite you. If you feel yourself getting obsessive about your lists, or fearful, drop them, sit back breathe deeply and relax, take a walk if you like and come back to them when you are calm and in a flexible more detached frame of mind. Remember to have fun, remember it is a game. As the Buddhists say: Non attachment.

The next step is to buy yourself a nice, bright poster board, and without cluttering it up, glue onto it pictures (from magazines or printed out from the internet) depicting your listed desires. Place affirmations for the fulfilment of these desires close to the relevant picture. Also in the middle of your poster board, it is essential to place a symbol of protection, this could be a picture of Buddha, a Holy Cross or an Angel. This gives your wants and wishes spiritual protection to help them manifest. View your picture board daily but keep it in a private place where others cannot see it, comment on it, ridicule it and thus possibly dissipate your wants and wishes with negativity. Do not worry about how you are going to make what is on your posterboard a reality, just enjoy daydreaming about it and follow any joyful, exciting, intuitive, even logical nudges in that direction. Thus you can cut through the confusion and accelerate your progress from where you are now to where you dream to be!

Many people describe confusing periods of their life as being those times when they felt like they were looking at life through a window, as if a huge piece of glass continually stood between them and the world. Never feeling that they are 'in the picture' but always an uncomfortable observer trying to create a sense of being connected and belonging. This can be a very frightening thing to face, but face it we must in order to dissolve that barrier between us and the world. Knowing that like all situations in life, the times of confusion come to teach us a lesson we need to learn. Explore finding out what that lesson may be by asking the simple question – What can I learn from this? To go with the flow, to trust, to feel my feelings more, to face my fears, to move house, to get a pet, to save money, to get a new job or training, to see a holistic therapist? What issue has this state of confusion highlighted for me, and what do I need to know or do in order to create order out of this confusion? See it as a positive process. Confusion is sometimes about living with the acknowledgement of the fact that surprise, surprise – We don't know it all! Learning to accommodate this realisation pushes us firmly towards the profound question – Well who or what am I going to trust to guide me, if I don't know everything, and the people around me also don't know everything? With a bit of luck the answer will urge you to find that inner guidance connected to Source Energy who does know everything because that Source Energy is within everything. It is within you, that is why your heart is beating.

Focus on one thing at a time. This uncluttered focus on one aspect of your life and what you want to achieve in that area of your life, is like a laser beam that cuts through confusion, and goes straight to the heart of the matter, the solution. Focus on the solution. Focus on what you want to achieve and take any step that seems to be going in that direction no matter how small and keep taking the next step, and the next, and the next, for it is often many, many, small steps that eventually lead to victory; often not quite knowing the next step until it reveals itself to you, in its own time and in its own way.

Affirmation: I get specific about what I want. I dwell and daydream about what I want. I am flexible in getting what I want. I trust my own inner knowing, I trust the perfect outworking of my life for the highest good of all concerned, with work I love and interesting pursuits in line with my preferences, ideals and standards.

**Recommended Reading**
The Purpose of Your Life by Carol Adrienne
One Day My Soul Just Opened Up Iyanla Vanzant

**Success and Failure**
Quote from the book Sathya Sai Baba The Embodiment of Love by Peggy Mason and Ron Laing – 'Many years ago we had a philosopher, Ralph waldo Emerson in the United States. He once was once asked, 'What is success in life?' He replied – 'To laugh often and much, to win the affection of children, to find the best in others, to endure the betrayal of false friends, to make the world a little better place to live in than when we were born into it, by rearing a little garden patch, improving some social condition, or helping a child grow healthier. To know that one life breathes easier since you lived. That is success."
I love that quote! Ponder it often, for it is quite different to the version of success we are given today to live up to. Material success is a hollow version and a false coin compared to real success as described above. So consider your priorities and what you feel success means to you personally. Is it amassing a lot of

money at any cost? Many people steal, or abuse animals (factory farming). Poison the fields with chemical fertilizers and pesticides (I know I came from a large arable farm in Ireland and witnessed it first hand). There will be Karma for those involved and though they may have for a while enjoyed great wealth, they suffered greatly in other areas of their lives. Was that really success, to act without conscience?

So, in comforting a child, making a friend laugh and doing a little poetry, gardening or volunteering with a genuine smile, working hard and blessing what you have, harming none, you are truly successful.

## Remember these thoughts:

Failure cannot live with persistence. Persistence produces results.

It's okay to make mistakes. Through mistakes we learn and grow.

Say to yourself – If you make a mistake don't worry, I still love and accept you just as you are, and you are changing, growing, learning all the time, for that you can be commended.

There is nothing like backing up to get a running start.

One who overcomes doubt and fear overcomes failure.

One should not take failure too seriously.

We rid ourselves of any feelings of unworthiness in order to achieve true and lasting success. As we go about our lives and find that even though we may try to move forward in a certain direction our way is blocked or riddled with setbacks. This could be for one of two reasons:

(a)     It could be a sign that you are going the wrong way and that this desire is not right for you. Time to reassess your true desires.

(b)     It could be a sign that there is a better way to accomplish your desires. These setbacks and failure experiences are teaching you to develop certain qualities such as tolerance, assertiveness, persistence or patience whilst you work toward your goal. They could be a sign that further education or study is needed.

Of course these are very subtle differences between (a) and (b). Only you can tell what your particular experience means. This does get easier as you learn to combine your intuitive and logical impulses.

An effective attitude to have if you feel like giving up, even though you know to persist would be a good idea, is this – I quit quitting! This is also a wonderful affirmation to push you into a positive frame of mind.

Affirm – I persist into slimness. I am getting slimmer and healthier every day. I am no longer a compulsive eater. I am a healthy eater. I love and accept my body now. I now lose excess weight permanently and naturally. I establish my own natural weight. I easily pinpoint and resolve my emotional issues. I no longer even crave food when I am physically full.

Success is the natural result of inner harmony. We have that inner peace and harmony when we are on top of our emotional issues and are aware of what we are dealing with emotionally, so to speak. Also reminding ourselves of a higher order, or divine unfoldment of your life, that Cosmic Plan or Life Purpose where certain challenges do have to be gone through and cannot really be avoided, but faced up to and resolved. Thus enabling you to mature, grow and become a different wiser, kinder, stronger person maybe. This is all part of the ability to create, or allow, order from chaos. So simply silently affirming – 'Divine right order is now established and maintained within my life and affairs. All is well' – is enough to (along with any logical steps to heal or improve the situation) help you during the time of transitioning out of the difficult and challenging, and into the peaceful and harmonious.

It really is like the Bible promise says – 'Seek ye first the kingdom of heaven and all these things shall be added unto you.' We gain everything we ever dreamed of, and even more, by turning within and achieving true success by following inner positive guidance and developing inner peace, harmony and divine order within our thoughts and emotions. Giving up compulsive eating and other addictions is, of course, part and parcel of achieving that sense of divine order and natural unfoldment.

When we feel peaceful and harmonious, ideas flow to us about how to develop our talents. We have the courage to follow those ideas. We simply do, no matter how scared or uncertain we may feel at times, for we, deep down, know it is the right thing to do albeit unconventional or scary. Looking back we realise it was simply logical and right to follow our own heart-felt desires and not be bullied or manipulated by others.

We follow our inner ideas and heart-felt nudges as to what to do, say or be. We see, through experience, what works. Life becomes more rewarding (albeit still a bit of a mystery). Life becomes more interesting and in line with our own personal goals, wants, needs and wishes. People of like mind appear in our lives, as we have the enthusiasm to do what we love, and dare to believe that we can be a success. We keep on keeping on and become (whether we realise it or not) an inspiration to others. Sure we ruffle a few feathers, but we easily and politely deal with those who are jealous or would hold us back for their own agenda.

So, may you persist into your own heart-felt success, be it to be a gardener, physicist, a lawyer, a painter or a home schooling mum, no matter what you desire to be – go for it!

Long term goals are accomplished by believing you deserve the best and by taking the small but necessary steps toward your goal. So, start now, taking the steps that enable you to transform your dreams into reality.

And what has this got to do with permanent weight loss? - You may ask. Well, fulfilling your life purpose, engaging in what you are interested in, and following your heart, is maybe what you have been avoiding for various reasons; and those reasons, and that avoidance of what you love, have left you with difficult and uncomfortable, maybe even painful emotions which you have suppressed with food when full. Stopping when full brought those emotions to light along with the unfulfilled needs behind them. Going for your heartfelt wants and wishes, has been the way to heal those painful emotions and thus no longer even crave to eat when full because of them. They have been healed, resolved, as emotional needs have been healthily met not unhealthily suppressed.

## Recommended Reading
They Dynamic Laws of Prosperity by Catherine Ponder Chapter 20
Creating Money Keys to Abundance by Sanaya Roman and Orin
Trust Your Intuition by John Dumais (audio)

## Loss and Disappointment
It could be the feeling of loss from the death of a loved one, or the unwanted break up of a relationship, a grown child leaving for college. It could be a feeling of abandonment left over from birth or childhood, a lack of parental love and understanding. Regardless of where it originated, along with allowing yourself to grieve, think in terms of forgiveness and Divine Restoration as a remedy for these feelings of loss and disappointment. For all that has seemed lost, can and is, being restored to you as you come into that frame of mind and consciousness through your own simple belief and faith in the possibility of that Universal Law of Divine Restoration.

This remedy works. Focus on being thankful. When you think about and write down all that you do have and are thankful for, it helps heal that sense of loss. This practice enables you to change your perspective from loss to gain. The natural cycle of life is that of birth, death and rebirth. Turn around those feelings of loss and disappointment through the idea of rebirth and restoration. Like a phoenix rising from the ashes, the natural healthy order of a life truly lived; and lived without turning to food when full, or drink, or drugs is all about rising from the ashes of the past, maybe even several times in one lifetime on one's road to improvement, healing and recovery.

Blessings and improvement, healing and recovery are in order don't block them by suppressing your sadness, fear and anger over losses when far greater good is in store for you. Allow painful feelings to flow. Feel the grief and let it pass for it does indeed pass. When you are overcome by the feelings of loss you maybe can repeat the Bible quote – 'I will restore to you the years which the locusts of lack hath eaten. Ye shall live in plenty and be satisfied.' I am not a particularly religious person but comfort often can be found in all the great Spiritual texts.

**Jealousy**

When you find yourself jealous of someone, ask yourself – What is this person achieving that I would love to achieve but feel I cannot possibly achieve?

What does this person have that I would also love to have that I consider impossible for me to have? Am I afraid that I will never have anything as wonderful as that?

When you are jealous or envious of someone, rather than suppress those feelings, thinking they are wrong, just notice them and realise that a part of you is saying – I would like something like that for myself, but I am afraid I will never achieve it.

Be aware that you cannot take from another what is rightfully theirs, but you can have your own equivalent. Jealousy has everything to do with fear. We all feel jealous when we are afraid that we will never be able to manifest our own version of what that other person has. It could be a successful career, a nice home, a car or a loving husband and genuine friends. Surely, we all desire these good things in life and we can all have what we desire when we take the necessary steps toward their achievement using various self-help manifestation skills, knowledge and intuition.

Feel your fear. Dissolve your fears by repeating positive affirmations about the attainment of your desire. Reassure yourself daily that you can have what you desire. No one loses. Look around and appreciate the simple everyday things you already have in your world and acknowledge that if you have already provided yourself with these things, then with the right thoughts, words and actions you can provide yourself with even more. Give yourself permission to expand, and have more of what you desire.

Everyone has their own success, their own relationships, special qualities and material goods. It is okay to want more and to be inspired by the qualities and possessions of another, for we too can aspire to such heights. Just decide and write down exactly what it is that you want and then ask yourself what is the first step toward the achievement of this that I desire? Then go about achieving that goal as best you can, believing that you can have it. Convince yourself that it is possible.

Jealousy also entails believing that you are depleted in some way because you are without that which you desire. Let us consider what this means as regards the desire to be slim. Most overweight women believe they are depleted because they are overweight. But I ask you this – Is your self-worth determined by your body size?

In order to deal effectively with jealousy you must acknowledge that you are not necessarily diminished in any way by carrying around however many extra kilos. You may see a slim woman and feel jealous. Feeling that you can never achieve slimness and feeling diminished because of your excess weight. You can think – It sure would be great to be slim. And you are right, it is great to no longer be a compulsive eater. But the reality of our slimmer sisters is actually a little different. A woman can be slim but bulimic, have low self-acceptance, and much self-loathing. A woman may be slim but suffer from alcoholism. A woman may be slim and recovering from a bad divorce. A woman may be slim but have cancer. This is reality. I do not know anyone fat or slim that is not working through some problem or issue in their lives. So why not realise that you are in no way diminished just because you are working through your particular problem, which happens to be a weight one. You are learning exactly what you need to learn at this moment in time. You are being challenged and it is true – when life goes well, it's a challenge, and when life goes badly – it's a challenge.

When you truly value yourself, and what you have, problems and all, releasing your fear of lack, planning towards and believing that you can have what you truly and honestly desire, you have little or no room for jealousy.

**Self-pity**

A feeling of loss, when indulged in could turn into self-pity, resentment and bitterness. Suppressing or indulging in feelings of self-pity is not generally considered healthy behaviour. Self-pity often masks sadness, grief or sorrow, in allowing yourself to feel your sorrow or grief you will automatically heal your self-pity.

Is pity the nearest thing to love that you got from a parent? 'Poor you' may have been all the love you received in many ways. Maybe you were ignored until something bad happened and then you got pity. Was pity better than nothing in terms of emotional nourishment, so that now it is the only emotional nourishment that you can give yourself? Ponder these things for in so doing you find the truth of your upbringing and how it is negatively effecting you today, and change it.

It is good to know some handy ways of breaking up those negative states of mind. Try allowing yourself to have a good cry with a box of tissues to help unblock that self-pity instead of suppressing grief and self-pity with food when full. Read Dr John Gray's book 'Mars and Venus Starting Over' for relationship issues. Forgiveness affirmation are also priceless in unblocking sadness, bitterness or resentment. The more you can feel your sadness and let it go, the healthier you will be and the more pleasant your life becomes.

Give yourself healthy self-acceptance and self-love instead of pity. Know you are strong in the face of challenging situations and do not crumble into self-pity and weakness. Take your time, learn new skills of personal empowerment and self-care and you will be able to change, become stronger and grow.

Visualise yourself in your present situation. Now visualise, if you will, how a person who is feeling sorry for herself would react in this situation. How would they act and react? How do they hold themselves and communicate? Are they successful? What opinions do the folk around her have about her? Is there any payoff in being this way in this situation? Gaining approval or sympathy for example?

Now I would like you to visualise how a self-assured, positive-minded person would approach the same situation. How would she feel, act and react? How are the others around her acting and reacting to her? Is her behaviour empowering or disempowering to her?

Now, which way do you wish to be in the world?

To also help with self-pity ask yourself – In what ways do I help me feel good about me? In what ways to I appreciate myself? In what ways do I validate, and nurture my very own skills and talents, likes and preferences?

## Guilt

Guilt is like a riverbank. When you feel guilty you are on that riverbank. When you flow with the river of life you do not experience guilt. You are at one with yourself and at peace with all. Your actions are in line with your own personal value system, you forgive yourself for any wrong you have done others in the past and acknowledge that you have learned the harsh lesson of what not to do, and you keep your actions kind to yourself and others. And if you can't be kind, you walk away. Neither inflicting harm nor allowing others to inflict harm on you, life moves on much more favourably.

Guilt is felt when we are not true to ourselves. Guilt is experienced when you allow an outer authority or person dictate to you against your wishes, wants or needs. In other words, we feel guilty when we do something we really do not want to do, often just to appease someone.

Ask yourself: What is it that I think I have done wrong? Forgive yourself. Reassure yourself that you are doing the best you can and resolve to never do that again if that is appropriate, and that you will do better next time. Know you can learn from mistakes.

Notice the issue of safety, for guilt has been described in the breathwork field as being the feeling that you have done something wrong in a world that is not safe.

Again self-forgiveness heals guilt. And reassure yourself that you can learn new patterns of behaviour especially when you feel guilty after a binge on food. It may be a time to delve into some self-help books or inspirational, spiritual You Tube Videos such as those of Ram Dass. A time of soul searching in order to clear out the pattern of eating when full and then feeling guilty about that overeating. This negative cycle can be broken, and having faith in your strength and ability to break a habit such as this, is empowering. This is establishing a new habit, a new eating pattern, a new way of relating to emotions and situations. Some say it is a lifelong endeavour of healing and growing in preference to the stagnation that is the suppression of feeling through eating when full.

**Rebirthing Discovery**

We know now that at birth we are completely conscious human beings. That means we feel, we think, we make conclusions.

Two midwives attended a lecture given by a pre- and peri-natal psychologist and Rebirthing Breathwork coach Binnie A Dansby. She asked the midwives that the next time they were around a woman giving birth, to guess what conclusions the new-born is making about the experience, considering the way she is being treated by the people present when she is born and shortly after. Well, they went away with this interesting idea in mind. When they came back to Binnie they commented on how much, doing that, had opened their eyes and helped them acknowledge that a lot of new born babies could make a lot of negative conclusions. They realised a gentler approach to birth is an urgent necessity.

I cannot stress this enough – babies are completely conscious and aware when they emerge from the womb. This extremely important fact is the major driving force in the great positive changes now occurring in the way babies are coming into the world.

Whilst attending a lecture in London by that same lady, the point I listened to with intent was that if we were born in hospital in the conventional way, involving the cord cut before it stops pulsing, separation from the mother, being weighed, measured and pricked, we could be carrying around deeply embedded negative conclusions about life. It is terrifying for a new born to be separated from her mother; traumatic for the mother too. In fact, in the book The Secret Life of the Unborn Child it has solid evidence that this often unnecessary separation causes 'the baby blues'. Pain, fear and guilt are feelings that result from this separation. Conclusions such as I am alone, life is painful, they don't like me, could be the result of being put in a plastic box next to mother instead of in being held her arms as nature intended.

There is no one here for me, I might die, no one is listening, I don't get my needs met, can be the result of being taken from mother, crying as a result of that separation and out of ear shot or maybe she is too drugged to respond. This is nothing less than emotional abuse. Thus deeply damaging negative thought patterns have been planted in the new born consciousness, laying a blueprint for life. Yes, the thoughts we have, those pre verbal conclusions we make, form the blueprint of our life. Because the medical profession does not recognise this, it goes un-noticed, and whether or not the parents have a say in this, is really up to the individuals involved. Hopefully many midwives and doctors are open to these important facts that must be considered and incorporated into the formula for a 'successful' birth.

We need to look at birthing practices as that which lay a foundation for the individual and collective life. When we look at our seemingly uncaring society, homelessness, addiction and war, we need to look deeply for causes and solutions.

So what! You may say – The baby is alive! Should we not be just thankful for that? Surely whatever the medical profession does is necessary? And yes a lot of what the medical profession does is necessary if you are talking about a broken leg or heart attack. But remember pregnancy and labour are not illnesses. And very few doctors or midwives know what a healthy natural birth looks like or could even stand to be in a room where one is occurring without freaking out due to their own unresolved birth trauma. This is where Rebirthing Breathwork comes in along with the work of Binnie A Dansby and Dr Fredrick Le Boyer author of Birth Without Violence and the pioneer in the natural birth / waterbirth movement.

The unfortunate thing is that most of us were born in the conventional way, carry birth trauma deeply embedded in our cellular memory, and have made deep-seated negative conclusions about life as a result of this birth imprint of weighing, separation and rough, unconscious handling by albeit well-meaning medical staff.

Whether or not you believe it, those original impressions about life that you made as you took your first breath, are deeply imbedded in you to this day, and effect your life and how you see the world. They form both the blueprint upon which your life is built, and a screen through which you see your life. That really means that whatever is in your subconscious mind helps create life as you know it.

Again the good news is that meditation, rebirthing breathwork, energy healing, affirmations, visualisations plus the Work of Byron Katie are all very effective tools to dissolve this deep seated negative programming from birth trauma, and clear up its present day negative unwanted effects. Thus allowing you to have positive conclusions about life and the power to mould and shape your life into a creation more to your liking. Be it a slimmer body, happier relationships or greater career and financial contentment this healing modality of clearing up birth trauma is certainly a major factor.

In closing: A new born who is born (as described in Part Two of Dr Fredrick Le Boyer's book Birth Without Violence) in a quiet dimly lit room, the mother moving about as her body dictates, with a tub of water there if she wishes to use it, pushing when she feels like pushing, in an upright position with the support she needs. A bean bag or the father there to catch the baby, delivered onto the mother's breast and cord cut only after it stops pulsing (usually about ten minutes) – that baby concludes - Life is kind, I am loved, I am safe, Life is sweet (breast milk is sweet) I am nourished, all is well. The life that naturally is created from that blueprint is a beautiful life.

**Stress and anxiety**

Stress and anxiety are the opposite of peace. When handled incorrectly these extremely uncomfortable states can prevent us from acting on our own behalf, leaving us feeling powerless and frustrated. Not a nice cocktail of emotions, and a cocktail that can cause many to eat when full and thus gain excess weight.

But a good way to deal with anxiety and stress is to develop their opposite – peace, until peace is the predominant feeling within our consciousness. Acting only on thoughts that come from a calm, grounded and peaceful state of mind is always a good idea. In tune with your own heartfelt desires and wishes, finding a way to create the life you want while healing your eating habit, moving and moving on becomes the order of the day, through emotions not suppressing emotions. Not thrown by setbacks or mistakes, keep moving and use reassuring thoughts and inner dialogue to create peace as you allow yourself to be born anew. Dropping the old anxious self we move away from what could actually be causing the anxiety – a violent or domineering spouse, parent or boss for example, you take control of what you can control, heal what you can heal emotionally within yourself and allow a better eating pattern, and life circumstance, prevail. Thus you become the empowered individual very much capable of acting on your own behalf.

Often we feel anxiety when we feel unwanted as children. When you find yourself feeling anxious ask yourself – Did I feel this way as a child? Try to recall a specific thing that left you feeling anxious – a parent who ignored you or overly criticised you perhaps? Allow deeper feelings and emotions to surface to simply be noticed, and understood and given space to be healed in the laser beam healing light of conscious awareness. They will dissolve, they will pass. Allowing yourself to really feel these emotions rather than suppressing them with food when full removes that which is standing between you and greater peace.

## Note - See Dr John Gray's book – What You Feel You Can Heal.

As we tune into our feelings and connect with our own true desires, we can also consider our own personal value system. Through this conscious awareness and conscious thinking we get to know what is truly right for us. What we desire does not always coincide with what others want from us. For example: your husband may want you to work full time but you want to be a stay at home mother. Or while living at home, your parents want you to become a lawyer and you want to study philosophy. Your sister in law may pressure you to come home and be your father's caregiver so she is not burdened with the job, but you do not want to, you prefer to stay away and continue to care for your own husband and children because you never got on well with your father.

We tend to feel anxious when we decide to go against our own personal value system; and also funnily enough, we can feel equally anxious when we go against what others want from us for fear of what they will do. People don't always like it when you stand up for yourself and your own values, but the important thing is that when you stand up for your own values there is an excitement and drive to stand your own ground that can delete any negative anxiousness that stems from the pressure placed on you by others. You can recognise where the anxiety is coming from, and in that clarity, simply carry on being true to your own heart.

We become more separate if you like, less dependent on the control freak's antics and attempts at manipulation. Often distancing ourselves from people like this, even cutting them out of our lives is necessary as we heal and grow and know what behaviour we will and will not tolerate from others. Life becomes more peaceful.

You become the healthy autonomous adult who considers and acts according to her own thoughts, feelings and values, even under pressure. You are less likely to role-play, adopt an uncomfortable stereotype, or conform to another's idea of who you 'should' be when your actions and words are in line with you own ideas of who you aspire to be and who you are.

Others may need us to fill a role or be a certain way, do certain things in order for them to feel in control. Doing what another wants us to do, when it goes against what we know to be right for us, is damaging and only leads to resentment and unhappiness on our part. Whereas, we can feel happy when our words and actions support our own personal value system. Often there can be tremendous pressure from others for us to maintain a certain role. Thus being yourself can be a tremendous challenge at times, but it is good to persist, as in the long run everyone benefits and relationships either dissolve (to make room for better ones) or improve. See my book My Life My Way, subtitle You Gotta Dig Deep in Order to Blossom available from Lulu on line publishing and Amazon.

Another important point I would like to make about anxiety is – not having an alternative way to deal with our unresolved feelings can cause anxiety when we first start to experience those feelings. This is why it is so important for us to find and use the healthy, alternative to eating when physically full as a means of dealing with our feelings. Thus we are not left 'high and dry' (anxious) when those feelings do in fact appear. Momentary eating when full at this time is quite normal.

As you already know, when we stop eating when physically full we are allowing the feelings with which we are uncomfortable, to emerge, so we can experience them again. This is a natural part of healing. However, if these feelings are too much for the recovering compulsive eater to experience, anxiety will take over and mask those uncomfortable feelings. Finding an easier way to experience these intense feelings clears up both the feelings and the anxiety. Often Rebirthing Breathwork is good to incorporate into one's life at this time, it really helps us feel, deal with, and integrate previously uncomfortable, even traumatic emotions. The Rebirthing Coach will be well versed in supporting you as you process your pain in the session. Another of John Gray's books is good here – 'How to Get What You Want and Want What You Have.'

For women especially anger is often felt to be unacceptable. It is childhood conditioning – girls don't get angry. The unhealthy and unnecessary suppression of a 'male' emotion in the young female. Now however, we are allowing all emotions to surface and come into our conscious awareness. If strong feelings of anger come up, we may be frightened by the strength of these emotions for we were never taught what they meant, or how to handle them in a healthy way. So subconsciously we distance ourselves from them through our severe unconscious judgement of the emotion called anger, and feel anxious instead, or experience anxiety intermingled with diluted anger. Resolving that feeling of anger, finding healthy ways to deal with anger such as beating the mattress or sofa, in private, with your fists, is the key to healing any anxiety related to that anger.
Anxiety can also stem from insecurity, which in turn stems from lack of love. Self-acceptance is a healing key here. Anxiety can also be linked to fear of failure and, funnily enough fear of success. Fear of the future can also be anxiety producing, and

can be dealt with through list making and planning – flexible planning and daydreaming in positive ways about the future while a reassuring self-dialogue can also help ease the anxious thoughts. Although anxiety can be described as extreme unease, it is somehow more tolerable than the original feelings of fear or anger that is masking it. Fear or anger may have 'triggered' the anxiety and therefore it is the fear and anger that must also be addressed, in order for the anxiety to not get to the stage where it renders you incapable of acting on your own behalf. So, the implementation of the various aforementioned tools is key.

Anxiety sometimes occurs when a woman becomes slim through dieting and starts to do all sorts of different things that she thought she would do slim, but never looked at the fears she might have around doing those new things – things her fat-self would never do. It is important to look at who we think we would be when we get slim. She may be a completely different person to who you are now with the excess weight. For example: As you are now, with the extra pounds, you might never go swimming, yet once you get slim decide that you can waltz around the swimming pool in a bikini totally unprepared for the unwanted attention you would get. So, preparing for the slim-you and the incorporation into your life the things you think you would do slim, into your life now, is essential as you become aware of all that the reality of being permanently slim entails. The resolving of these issues (such as unwanted attention) is an essential part of becoming your slim-self and being happy with that size and shape and the activities you do or do not do. The emotional resolving allows the slim figure you attain to be permanent.

You may subconsciously equate being slim with wearing a bikini and tons of confidence, but discover the reality is you feel vulnerable, uncomfortable and exposed. The healing will be to allow your slim-self be a person who wears a one-piece swim suit, with a towel or sarong nearby to cover up when you feel the need. You may have thought 'covering up' was only for the overweight-you, so allow the security of what the overweight you does to be brought into what the slimmer-you does. Fat or slim you are doing what suits you and works for you personally. This is empowerment. This is no longer letting a body size dictate what you wear or do.

## Peace

'The blessing of living from the eternal perspective is the accomplishing of inner peace.' This quote from the Seer Almine Barton is very profound in my opinion, for to attain 'living from the eternal perspective' would be quite an achievement to say the lease. First of all what exactly does it mean to live from the eternal perspective? To my understanding it is a bit like seeing the big picture, knowing that whatever disturbs your inner peace can and is surrounded, overpowered and obliterated by some benevolent perspective that allows peace.

To attain a peaceful frame of mind is so valuable. Most people already know this but seek peace as if it were some illusive quality which seems impossible to attain. There are also those who dislike peace intensely, consciously or subconsciously, allowing drama be an integral part of their lives. That drama distances them from the underling painful emotions that need resolving. These people somehow feed off this drama, making many their victims. Those who seek peace however must realise that it is not under the control of some outside force – if only he'd change, if only the world would change then I would feel peaceful. But it does not work like that. It does not come from money either, or being a certain weight. No, rather it can be attained through meditation, and emotional resolving.

**Tools to help attain peace:**
If you find yourself living with people who provoke arguments or are negative and critical you may need to seriously consider moving. Only you can really judge your living situation and decide what is best for you. Eating when full to dull the pain of a bad environment that you wish to leave and grow out of, is not the answer. Being fully aware of the pain your living conditions are causing you, is essential for you to plan your escape out of them.

In a relaxed moment dwell on the phrase – I am peace, I am tranquillity, I am. Enjoy the luxurious feel of such words as serenity, comfort, light and love. Conjuring up these feelings and allowing yourself to melt into them so to speak, you are allowing yourself to become a magnet for a more peaceful life.

Bring plants into your life, into your home or office if you can. And get out into nature as much as you can. A gentle walk in nature is very peace inducing. Or sit in your garden if you are too tired from a long work shift for example.

Cut out beautiful pictures from a magazine or print them out. Paste them into a note book or keep them in a folder to look at when stressed. This can shift you attention to peace.

If you are working on a problem. Physically relax. Either with your eyes closed or focusing on a plant or flower appreciating it, allow your eyes to go a little out of focus and affirm – The perfect idea that can heal this situation is coming to me now. I am open and receptive to the perfect solution to this issue. The perfect solution is in my mind, I access it now. My problems are solved easily and in peace.

Be non-attached to the outcome, just follow your own ideas, your joy, do what you are interested in and follow what interests and excites you. Go as far as you can with it and then, when you can go no further, seek the next healthy thing in your life that draws your attention, interest and excitement. This is the direction you can go in life to attain your goals.

Non-attachment to the outcome is necessary for it opens the way for what you want to be delivered to you in ways you never could have imagined. See You Tube videos of Daryl Anka the channel for Bashar for further information on this subject.

The concept of Divine Order is also a helpful one. If we feel stressed or anxious, affirming Divine Order is soothing and allows us to see things with a new more positive perspective.

After all, major growth comes out of chaos. So do not fear the chaos but affirm Divine Order as you follow your bliss. We cannot control many things in our lives but the concept of Divine Order reassures us that there is a benevolent presence at work in our lives and it is always trying to show us the highest solution to any given problem or situation. Everything in our lives is there for a good reason. We are to learn an important and unique lesson from having gone through the experience. Once we have learned what the given situation is teaching us, that situation or problem either transforms or disappears and we move on in life. Remember the age-old truth – Life never punishes. It teaches.

Maybe, if you look back on the various challenges that life has given you in the past, you may realise that after they passed you learned some valuable lesson, you became stronger or discovered some inner resource such as compassion which had lain dormant before that challenge came into your life. May be a chunk of inner healing occurred through facing that challenge. Spend some time now and consider those times. Acknowledge and appreciate yourself for your ability, courage and strength. Affirm – I am in Divine Order now. My life is in Divine Order now. Everything is in Divine Order now and everything is working out for the highest good of all concerned.
Before going to sleep at night repeat to yourself – I am loved, I am in the love of peace. Tomorrow will be a good day.

## List making and planning

This is particularly good if you want to become more organised. It can also help with feeling overwhelmed, fearful of the future or want to make changes in your life. It can be used as an everyday tool to aid daily living.

**The 'I don't want this' list:** Simply list everything you no longer want in your life, such as your financial lack or your weight problem. Then after each write – 'This is fading out of my life as I learn the lessons it brings. This is now healed and eliminated from my life.

Then make a list of what you do want in your life – The 'I'd like that!' list: List everything you would like to manifest in your life. After each listed desire write – 'I have faith that his or something better now manifests for me in perfect ways at the perfect time.' Such as a better job or training. A good relationship and genuine friends.

And then simply list all things you are grateful for in your life, your health, your house, your job for example. The fact that you can breathe, walk and talk, simple things like that.

The purpose of the first list is a cleansing and releasing one. When we write down a list of things we do not want in our lives and after each one write - This too is fading from my life – what we are in fact doing is giving the mind a very clear, strong and definite message of clearance. First we write the problem and then the elimination message. Thus feeding the brain the idea that the problem is definitely on its way out, fading and being eliminated. Because of the way the mind works, much like a computer, what you repeatedly feed it, is what it produces in terms of feelings ideas and results. The planting of a seed of a problem fading creates the fading of that problem. The writing down and even visualising what is on your 'I want' list quickens the manifestation of that desire. Do not worry about how these desires or wants are going to come about, you are an unlimited spiritual being with the power to create good in your world and the tool of visualisation is a key that unlocks your creative power for manifesting that good. Only visualise good for yourself and others, for what you send out comes back to you multiplied so be sure to send out good and thus you shall receive!

Author and originator of Quantum Healing Hypnosis Technique (QHHT) Dolores Cannon stated 'Earth is a school where we learn about emotions and limitation.' This is so true, and many of us have learned how to deal with our emotions through suppressing them, distancing ourselves from them through eating when full or other addictions. We, through experience, realise that that way of dealing with emotions only causes excess weight and the remaining unresolved emotional issue still bothering us. Nothing got resolved or healed, no lesson was learned, no wisdom gleaned. With this perspective we can easily start seeking the alternative. So, as you give up eating when full and become more used to feeling your feelings, both pleasant and unpleasant, you can practice developing pleasant feelings from within and unpleasant feelings dealt with by asking yourself – Given the fact I feel this way (sad, depressed, lonely, angry, frustrated or fearful for example) what would I like to do now? How can I improve this situation? What is this feeling telling me about this person or situation? Is there any action I can take to improve this, or can I just 'sit with' this intense feeling and allow it to pass?

Ask yourself often – What emotion am I experiencing right now? Thus you practice getting and staying in tune with your emotions.

Breathe deeply as you turn inward. Notice if the emotion is located somewhere in your body. You can tune inwards and become aware of your emotions almost anytime and anywhere; when you are doing the washing up, walking the dog, watching television. The more often you tune into your feelings, the more familiar you will become with being aware of and comfortable with your feelings and subtle energy system.

Focus on your belly – your solar plexus, diaphragm area when you are around other people. This is your area of emotional receptivity from your surroundings and people. If you are around someone who is suppressing their feelings you could 'pick up' on those feelings, and end up 'holding them' in that area. If too much of their suppressed emotion gets into you, you could start acting it out, getting angry or sad for example. The phrase 'That person really got to me' is referring to this dynamic, this invisible exchange of energy and emotion, which is transferred via both what they say, their tone of voice and their actual presence close to you. So distancing yourself from them is one of the first healing tools to use.

Another way to protect your solar plexus is to fill yourself up with golden light, feel it spill out of you and rest around you like a bubble, and then imagine mirrors <u>facing away from you</u> and towards the other person. This will simply mirror back to the person themselves, whilst protecting you from their unresolved emotional gunk. Remember it is very important to have the mirrors facing towards the other person – it is their own reflection that they need to see.

You can instead imagine a disc of white light directly in front of your solar plexus, like a shield protecting you.

Ask yourself often – Am I physically hungry right now? Am I physically full or somewhere in between, like peckish? These are ideal questions to ask yourself often as you try to change your eating habits. It gives you practice turning inward and becoming more aware of your body's own sensations of genuine physical hunger and genuine physical fullness.

Think a little bit more deeply about the things you are inclined to take for granted and say a silent 'thankyou' to all the people who are part of the food that you eat, from the food server to the factory worker, to the farmer. Think about who made the clothes you wear, send them a silent prayer of prosperity and joy in their life, good health, good working conditions and pay. Really grasp all that occurred to create the physical reality that is yours.

## Divine Inspiration

Look up these bible quotes if you are ever in need of some divine inspiration:

Psalms 37:1, Psalms 46:1, Psalms 119:66, Psalms 73:24
John 14:27, John 14:1, John 10:10, Luke 18:27, Luke 17:21
Mathew 11:28, Mathew 7:7, Romans 8:31, Philippians 4:8 – 23
Proverbs 3:5, Mark 11:24, Ephesians 6:13, James 5:16

## Security and Flexibility

There is great healing power to be found in nature. Many of you already enjoy time in nature, taking regular walks, and even if you live in a city the park can provide an escape from the cold concrete of city life. Spending a lot of time indoors on our computers or phones is also to be balanced with time outdoors, gently walking, jogging, playing tennis if you enjoy sports or simply sitting in the garden reading a book or meditating. It is of vital importance for you to evaluate how much time you spend outdoors and really judge for yourself whether or not you need to increase it. Breathing in fresh air, being aware of your surroundings and allowing yourself to sit and gaze at a tree or bush until you feel peaceful and even at one with its life force energy. In James Redfield's classic book The Celestine Prophecy he talks about the auras around plants and how we can all easily see them with a little gazing and relaxation. There is also a Buddhist 'Walking Meditation' that one can adopt at times to allow greater peace and mindfulness into one's life throughout this journey of personal growth and becoming slim.

We must remember the power of nature, that the aspects of every plant are different and can help us. Every plant is a medicine of which Aromatherapy, Bach Flower Remedies, Herbalism and Homeopathy are proof. Their work is gentle yet strong and we can tap into it through the above therapies.

## Visualisation

This is a beautiful visualisation to help you feel grounded yet flexible. Trees are the epitome of this, their roots go deep into the earth creating stability for the overground growth of swaying flexible branches and fluttering leaves. They give us oxygen so their importance is phenomenal.

Coming from a place of self-acceptance, love, guided through wisdom, experiencing our own unique sense of self, knowing what we want, feeling grounded and flexible as we go about getting it, we feel secure. The tree is the perfect symbol of the higher self. It draws its nourishment from both mother earth and father heaven. Standing strong and mighty between the two. (Do not do this visualisation when driving or operating machinery)

Sit in a comfortable position and I would like you to close your eyes and relax. Now, from where you are sitting, place your feet firmly on the floor, I would like you to imagine you are a tree… Feel your roots going deep into the ground… feel your network of roots providing you with stability and balance… Allow your roots to go deep, very deep. You can sway gently and they support you… When you feel your roots can go no deeper, feel them finding ways around rocks, even having the power to go through rocks, finding weakness in the rock and finding water and nourishment deep, deep in the earth, unknown territory to those who merely dwell on the surface… Feel your roots anchoring themselves comfortably in the deep earth… Feel the refreshing water being pulled up through the root system through the trunk and into the branches and leaves experiencing the glory of the sunshine and moonlight alike… Feel the stillness, the timelessness of you as a nature being… feel all things changing around you… for you live for hundreds of years, simply solid yet flexible, giving shelter to those who sit beneath your branches, feel them love your beauty, hug your trunk and wonder at your age and grace. Feel the rain on your leaves, branches and trunk, washing away all you do not want… Feel the flourish of your autumn colour, the fading golds and browns… the ease of letting them go in winter… the strength that can withstand snow and wind… Feel the joy as you burst forth new buds awakened by the sunshine of Spring and the relief of fulfilling your life purpose, connected to the moon phases and movement of stars overhead, the light and the dark, the seasons and the air… The water flowing through you and on you, the warm summer breezes around you… cleansing… healing… you are one with nature… Enjoy this scene as long as you wish and then slowly let the scene fade… be aware of your breathing… and gently come back to your room, become aware of yourself sitting on the chair, your feet on the floor, your back against the back of the chair and gently open your eyes, yawn and stretch.

There are several things that enable us to feel secure. One is a strong sense of self, the other is our sense of connection to whatever it is we regard as our Ultimate Source. This is sometimes called God, Spirit, Universal Intelligence, Allah or Buddha, Divine Love, the Divine Mother or simply the positive overcoming power of the human spirit.

I also believe strongly that our sense of self is greatly dependent upon how self-accepting we feel. Self-approval is also a necessary requirement for a strong sense of security. If we were ignored or criticised a lot in childhood, if we were not spoken to with love or acceptance we will grow up feeling insecure, for intuitively we know we must be accepted and loved in order to be cared for properly. We may even feel we do not have a right to exist. And as many of these feelings become subconscious, or so 'normal' we don't even notice them, it can cause even more problems. As we give up our habit of eating when full these are some of the things that may come to light, and developing self-acceptance is the answer as is explained earlier in this book. So, self-acceptance, self-love, and security are pretty much inseparable. If you did not get that all important love and approval from your parents or caregivers in childhood, it is extremely important for those past wounds to be healed and a healthy self-acceptance and self-love be established in order for you to increase (or establish) your feelings of security.

In adulthood, having a sense of self, an awareness of your connection to Source, knowing what you want and being able to be assertive and firmly but lovingly communicate with others, leads to your real needs being met, and thus your personal, psychological and physical security is provided.

**What would I do now if I knew I could not fail?**
In other words - What would you do if you knew success was guaranteed? Write down, between three and ten different things; for example, write a book, go back to college, learn to paint, have a child, home-school your child, seek another job with more pay and better working conditions, leave your current job, marry, divorce, or move to the country.

Look at your answers. Circle one and write down three or more steps you could take to help yourself accomplish it. Circle one of those steps and do it this week. With things such as write a book, the writing can be done for one hour daily with weekends off. Or looking for a new job can be done for an hour each evening. Jogging can be done three times a week for example, for fifteen minutes. Use your own judgement to create a new schedule and habit that is ultimately life changing through taking these small steps.

**Five pounds joyous spending!**
Imagine you are given five pounds for the sole purpose of spending joyously – what would you spend it on? Remember

this is joyous spending! For example you could buy a colourful ribbon or a small crystal, a perfumed soap or pretty notebook or pen.

If you can spend a small amount of money joyously then you will also get pleasure from larger amounts. If however, you find it difficult to spend a small amount joyously, then larger amounts will not give you pleasure, for you will not have learned how to spend joyously. So, the lesson to be learned is – Practice spending your small amount joyously for there are many rich people who really do not do that. They spend to feel better, it is a compulsion, and any 'feeling better' is short lived, they do not always spend wisely, or help people they know are less well off. They have no generosity of spirit for they are not coming from an emotionally full place themselves, even though they may have all the material items that many would consider happiness producing.

**Ask yourself** – Is there something bothering me? Is something concerning me? Something I am worried about, or feel is a problem? If the answer is no, then allow yourself to feel grateful about that fact. However, if the answer is yes, then ask yourself - How can I heal this, how can I view this in a more positive way so it gets healed? And what is the lesson I could learn from this? What is the issue – lack of trust, lack of love or commitment, approval or respect? How can I give me more of that lacking quality?

**A note on the power of the mind** – Whatever you regularly picture in your mind, or hold in your imagination you can have, in reality, in your life! This sure puts day dreaming in a different light! So get busy visualising in detail the kind of life you would like to have. This practice not only helps you alter and change your life for the better, but helps you see clearly what might stop you from altering and changing your life for the better. Visualising a goal helps you to recognise any subconscious defeat thoughts or belief systems, which may be sabotaging your good efforts. When you think about and visualise a desired goal, often you feel fear or doubt as you visualise a certain detail of the desired goal. This is your half-hidden negativity around having that goal, and potentially can stop your manifestation in its tracks if given any credence. The negativity can be thought through and resolved, sorted out and dealt with in the realm of the imagination. It is the avoidance of facing and resolving that negativity that has often caused us to subconsciously avoid actualising our dearest goal. In other words our subconscious fear can actually cause psychological blocks which prevent us attaining our goals. Regularly visualising the positive changes you want to see actualised in your life is the way to uncover any such blocks, doubts and fears, bringing them to your conscious awareness to be resolved. A goal is much easier to realise once the conscious and subconscious concerns around that goal have been looked at and delt with appropriately. As regards losing excess weight and becoming slim, we visualise ourselves slim and stay with the visualisation or repeat the visualisation enough to unearth the previously hidden fears of being the slim attractive woman. We then consciously address those fears, find ways of healing those fears so that we can become slim and be able to handle the things we were unconsciously afraid of, such as unwanted attention, or jealousy from other women.

Once you have faced your doubts and fears you may find you have a feeling of acceptance of the visualised results. A feeling that it is possible to accomplish what you once thought of as only a dream that you wished could come true.

You can have those positive desired dreams. The results you visualise or something even more appropriate can come to you as you persist to work in this inner way. Inner preparation, coupled with appropriate action fuelled by positive thoughts and feelings, creates improved outer results.

## A work of art

Regard your body as you would a work of art. View it as such! If you are critical of your body and do not accept its size and shape completely, then you can use this simple technique to help you develop greater self-acceptance. Why? Because self-acceptance and change go hand in hand. Yes, the attitude of self-acceptance actually helps you change that which you are so reluctant to accept now. Accepting an overweight body means you understand how it got that way - through suppressing emotional issues via eating when full, and it, and you, are innocent. You are in the process of changing that which 'got it that way' and now you are preparing for the slimmer version of you.

So, the next time you are in front of a mirror, try sending out thoughts and feelings of acceptance and appreciation. View your reflection as a work of art. Maybe even a work of art that you do not really like but are trying hard to appreciate. Notice your curves. Cease judging and criticising. Just look, appreciate, consider the subtle shading which the light creates on your face and form. Notice how your clothes fit. Are they baggy or tight? Notice the colour and tone of your skin. Just look without judgment. If there is judgement just notice that too, and realise that you can choose another more positive, self-accepting attitude. Whose voice is in your head? Your mother's? Your father's? Forgive them if they criticised, they were wrong and you can choose to be of a different frame of mind now. Focus on appreciating your body. Do this over the next few weeks and months until a totally self-accepting friend looks back at you.

## Nature and healing

Feelings are like clouds floating in the sky. Acknowledge them as they pass by for they are passing by. They came to pass not to stay. By eating when full though, we make them stay. By feeling them – they pass, they heal, they do not bother us once healed, they do not trigger us into our addictions, once healed. Feeling them, heals them. Feeling the intensity of the emotional issue, helps heal the emotional issue.

Addiction is a weed. Suppression is it's root. When you eliminate the root you eliminate the weed permanently.

Affirmations, like a river work sometimes rapidly, sometimes slowly. As a river flows it churns up and deposits sediment on the river bed and banks, leaving the water flowing forward, and later, clean, clear, calm pools can form. As we work with affirmations, our feelings are flowing through us, sometimes churning up negative emotion in order to clear it out, allowing us to leave behind negative thoughts and feelings so that we can ultimately be clean, clear and moving forward, eventually meeting our own calm places of inner and outer peace.

As we travel through life shedding negative feelings easily and in peace through forgiveness and emotional release, old, negative experiences become the fertile soil out of which our new good grows. We must seek that seed of goodness – the positive in the flood of negative feelings and experiences – acknowledge it's presence, make sure it gets plenty of 'positive thought' sunshine and give ourselves a well-deserved pat on the back as that positive seed grows blossoms and bears fruit.

A goal or a dream is like a flower. Water it, make sure it gets the light, the right temperature and moisture it requires, and simply allow it to grow and blossom.

## Criticism

Criticism, either self-criticism or being critical of other people or things, is detrimental. It leaves us feeling negative and in a low frame of mind; certainly not conducive to good health, relationships and well-being. Being over critical could also contribute to, or even cause arthritis, as stated in this quote from the book Heal Your Body by Louise L Hay. 'Arthritis: Probable Cause – Feeling unloved. Criticism, resentment. Healing affirmation: I am willing to release the pattern in my consciousness that created this. I am love. I now choose to love and approve of myself. I see others with love.'

So steer clear of being critical, or if you find you must judge others, take a look at Byron Katie's free worksheet called 'The judge-your-neighbour worksheet' from www.byronkatie.com or www.thework.com It turns our criticism of others into a self-healing tool and helps you develop a self-accepting, kinder attitude toward yourself and your fellow human.

Criticism is a bad habit and repetition of new positive ideas about how you want your life to be, instead of complaining and criticising how it is, will help you alter and change from within out the experience you have of life. Start practicing the new habit of acceptance and praise. When we stop being critical of others and ourselves it allows us to feel good about ourselves, boosting our self-confidence, and genuine self-esteem in a healthy non-egotistical way.

Start by quietly noticing your thoughts. Try forgiving those of whom you are critical, send them as much compassion and even love if you can. You don't have to be in their presence, in fact if they were abusive to you it is best to send that compassion and forgiveness from a distance, a great distance. I personally put the Irish Sea between me and my family of origin!

Whenever you catch yourself thinking a critical or resentful thought about a person, stop, and turn your thinking around and send them thoughts of pity or compassion if you cannot muster love and forgiveness. And remember: A thought of forgiveness goes a long way to healing _you_.

## Energy and fatigue

A lot of people think that they will automatically have more energy once they are slim. However there is more to feeling energetic than losing excess weight.

It takes a lot of energy to suppress a feeling or emotional issue. Once we start experiencing our feelings rather than suppressing them, then we have all that energy for our own positive use. Feeling and experiencing our feelings is energising for us. Suppressing our feelings depletes our energy. Doing what we do not want to do, depletes our energy, and saps our spirits. Doing what we do not want to do makes us feel tired whether fat or slim.

Have a goal that you genuinely feel enthusiastic about, create a plan for achieving it – this is energising. Bringing love to what you do (even if it is not ideal) while working towards your goal, is energising. Stay away from people who sap your energy. And needless to say hard work with naturally make us feel tired whether we are fat or slim.

Shallow breathing tires us. Shallow breathing also keeps us distanced from our feeling. Good deep breathing, when outdoors especially energises us and also helps us stay with and integrate our emotions. Although it is tiring to carry around excess weight, being slim in and of itself does not ensure extra energy. So do not be too surprised or disappointed if you become slim and still feel tired, it could be many factors contributing to that, and at that point in time it will be appropriate to heal them. Just remember – Do you never see a tired slim woman?

Resolving and integrating uncomfortable or painful feelings does ensure extra energy, and the loss of excess weight that has been gained as a result of eating when full to suppress those feelings.

The type of food we eat does affect our energy levels, so you can experiment with that if tiredness becomes an issue when slim. Also cutting out alcohol can give us extra energy. And doing a good quality detox can also help energy levels.

When you are feeling tired, ask yourself: Am I really tired or do I want to sleep in order to avoid my feelings? If you are really tired, then sleep. Have a nap if you can. One or two hours in the afternoon or early evening is great, and you may then find that as little as four to six hours sleep is enough at night when you are napping daily. Just experiment and listen to your body, you will fall into rhythm with its own needs.

If however you think you are sleeping because you have an emotional issue that you want to run away from (buying into the idea that when you wake up it will be gone) then check in with your feelings and ask the magic question – 'Given the fact I feel this way what would I like to do now?' And follow up on the healthy appropriate response.

Basically, the equation we have here is:
Resolved Emotional Issues equals Increased Ability to Stop Eating When Physically Full, Energy Flowing plus Natural Permanent Weight Loss.

## Healing Attitudes

Peace, joy and comfort are to be found in positive attitudes, or as I like to call them healing attitudes. Problems in and of themselves are never insurmountable. It is our attitudes towards these problems that make them either insurmountable or easily solved. This means, that the power to overcome is in our attitudes toward whatever life may be confronting us with, rather that the problem itself.

Can our attitudes really help us overcome our problems, rather than feeling like a victim of them? The answer is yes! Whatever your problem, feel the feelings involved and apply the healing balm of a positive attitude, thus empowering yourself to overcome that problem as you do. A simple affirmation that I learned from Catherine Ponders book The Dynamic Laws of Prosperity is – 'Something good will come from this, things are getting better and better for me now.' Or the classic 'Every day in every way things are getting better and better for me now'. I like to also put the words 'I have faith that…' before each of those affirmations. I have faith that every day in every way things are getting better and better for me now.

Start developing a positive attitude by calling your problem a challenge and calling any fear a concern. It helps dissipate any strong emotional charge, and helps you find solutions, so you can move through the challenges and concerns of life which we all have. Have faith that you can meet this challenge successfully and after you have dealt with that challenge effectively, you will be stronger and wiser. Our challenges are needed opportunities for us to grow, painful though they may be, it is in meeting and healing them that we find peace.

As the old song says accentuate the positive. It is a very simple way to help you accomplish much and the good news is anyone can do it, it is free. A positive thankful frame of mind makes you feel good. Try this – Before going to bed every night take a note book and pen (or your phone) and write down all the positive things that happened to you that day. Also write down all the things you are thankful for, all the things that went well for you that day and allow yourself to feel thankful for all you have taken for granted. Running water, the food, the job, the friends, the health and the blue sky above.

For whatever you want more of in your life, create an affirmation of thankful increase, for example, if you want more money an affirmation of thankful increase would go something like this – I give thanks for an increased financial income for my own personal use, every week now. If you want more love in your life – I give thanks for increased love in my heart and in my life.

Yes this does mean that you are giving thanks for what you desire before you actually get it or see it in your life. You are giving your desire a sure vote of confidence that it shall appear. Exercising your faith if you like. Faith is as strong a force in the universe as love. Like a magnet, giving thanks before you see the outer manifestation of your desire, you draw it to you mystically, magically and practically. So, you now know a new method for altering and changing your life, moulding and shaping it into a life more to your liking, but like any art or skill it must be practiced and mistakes allowed in order to master it – try it out for yourself and experiment with the tools now given to you to use.

**Psychological blocks**

At some stage in our personal growth we all experience a psychological block. This is when we know what to do, but we are unable to do it. Self-sabotage, it is also known as. This is usually due to fear, anxiety or lack of trust. It manifests as a feeling of not being able, not being ready, or not even wanting to take the next step to aid our own self-improvement. It could involve, not having the time or energy to take the required action which would enable us to move forward and improve. External circumstances can actually stop us, or seem to stop us, and often frustration is the order of the day.

So how can we deal effectively with our psychological blocks? Well, first and foremost go easy on yourself! Psychological blocks are a sign that you have already moved forward in your life. So much so, that you bumped into one! Often there is a temptation to criticise ourselves. After all, here we have positive proof that our best attempts have not managed to shift that frustrating blockage. This is, in truth a very inaccurate way of looking at such a block. Remember, we have had enough of self-condemnation and criticism. Refrain from self-blame! Yes, refrain from entertaining such a harmful, wasteful and harsh frame of mind. The truth is, you are doing fine and getting better all the time. Sometimes, the reality of personal development is three steps forward and two steps back. Allow yourself to continue with the good work, remembering to really acknowledge even the smallest sign of improvement.

The practice of self-forgiveness, is all you need to remember and focus on, where guilt and self-condemnation about psychological blocks are concerned. If you have a block with the practice of forgiveness and cannot forgive yourself then I suggest you just continue to be blocked, continue to condemn yourself, but be aware and conscious of what you are doing until you wake up to the detrimental effect you are having on yourself and your desire to hurt yourself because you feel guilty; continue until you get so bored or ill that you realise you are not helping yourself or anyone else. You will eventually find the strength and willingness to forgive yourself and know you deserve that forgiveness and self-understanding. Even putting forth the smallest effort can bring a breakthrough. It is always worth putting in effort and persisting. It is okay if this only happens after life has dealt you a blow so strong that the fright pushes you into action!

We cannot afford the luxury of a negative thought, is so true and many of us learn this truth through our experiences of our own personal growth, of which becoming permanently and naturally slim is part. All in all, it is always just a matter of going easy on ourselves whilst persistently exploring and resolving our fears of both accomplishing our goals, and our fears of things getting worse.
Wallowing in the block can be a good thing, as long as it is a short wallow with conscious awareness of what we are doing. Without condemnation use what strength you can muster to start to take the necessary steps to dissolve the blocks for good.

If it is a feeling of extreme anxiety or sorrow that is blocking you, it is your inability to feel that extent of anxiety or sorrow that drives you back to the old habit of eating when full to numb yourself. However you can, in time, dissolve the block by doing clearing exercises instead of eating when full. There are many to choose from. You can book a session with a local energy healer or therapist you feel drawn to work with. A holistic healing workshop, AA, a support group or good friend can help you gain a higher perspective on any feelings or emotional issues you feel at the mercy of; and through keeping a higher perspective, the block can always be chipped away at until totally dissolved over time. Thus leaving you free to move into a better healthier way of life.

Here is an affirmation for helping us attain that higher perspective and dissolve blocks: I am an unlimited spiritual being, full of light, love and the ability to do any good thing to heal myself. All my psychological blocks are dissolving in perfect time, in the perfect way. I am balanced, healthy and free. I move forward and claim my good results safely and in peace.

**About doubts**

Do you doubt your ability to succeed? If you doubt that you can do it, achieve your goal, make the career change, get the education or overcome the eating disorder and lose excess weight permanently, then make it your job to convince yourself that you can do it!

Set yourself the task of dissolving your doubts and fears. Fear is usually behind all our doubts. Feel your fear, face your fear and the doubt can vanish. Begin to have faith in yourself and what is possible for you to achieve. Healing your problems with food is very possible for you as is becoming slim. Try these following exercises:

Write out: I cannot heal my eating disorder because… (e.g. I have never been able to do so in the past)

Now change it around to – I can heal my eating disorder because even though I have failed in the past I can succeed now. I am sure if even one other person in the world has managed to heal their eating disorder, I can too. I can constantly learn the finer points of why I eat this way and how to alter and change my eating patterns to those of a naturally slim person.

Notice your thoughts and change them into their positive opposites, play with the wording until you find a life-enhancing healing formula of positive words that fuel your further growth away from addiction to food when full and into your slim-self!

You can also add phrases like: With the help of God / Angels / my higher power. With the help of 'All That Is Good' I can succeed in healing myself of the craving to eat when full. Other women have succeeded and so can I. Today is a new day. I forgive myself for past failures gleaning the lesson of that experience I become wiser. I now claim my good health. I now allow healthy eating patterns evolve through emotional resolving, eating when genuinely hungry and stopping when genuinely full. I mentally and emotionally learn to accept my slim self now. My own naturally slim body emerges at the right time in the perfect way. I become permanently and naturally slim easily and in peace.

**Now complete the following sentences:**
I can heal my eating disorder because…
Example: There are many books written on this subject and they are showing me how it can be done. Such as 'When Food Is Love' And 'Why Weight? A guide to ending compulsive eating' by Geneen Roth. And 'Fat Is A Feminist Issue' by Susie Orbach. Naturally Slim by Dr Cherie Martin. I can study these books.

I can lose weight permanently because…
Example: Other women using these non-diet methods have achieved natural permanent weight loss and so can I. I could start a local study group around one of these books for support and guidance.
I can remember the phrase - One who overcomes doubt and fear, overcomes failure. I can reassure myself that I can succeed. I can remember my past successes, big and small. I can take the time to really acknowledge those successes and congratulate myself. The more I am able to acknowledge my past successes the easier it is to accomplish new ones.

**Guidelines for a self-help support group**
The individual within the group can make enormous breakthroughs in terms of realisation, enlightenment and resolving what was once a problem or unresolved emotional issue. The sharing of experiences, support and focus on solution finding is a very dynamic way to tackle a problem and heal it

completely. It actively allows women to find and experience what life is like as a healed compulsive eater.

**Guidelines:**

No smoking, eating or drinking alcohol during the group meeting.

**Be focused and to the point:** Keep to important and significant points. Do not waste time with distractions or too many unimportant details.

**No trivia:** No talking about the weather or the latest news or gossip. Keep on track. Lots of sentences starting with – 'I feel… I felt… The issue I am dealing with now is… I overate when… That binge I had was to do with… My relationship with… is making me overeat. When I felt like a binge on chocolate and I asked myself - What feeling is this? – I realised I felt… And when I asked myself - Given the fact I feel this way, what would I like to do now? I decided to…

You see how this type of focus will really help you unravel your issues with food, size and shape? You see, this way we are getting straight to the point, and starting collectively and individually to focus on possible solutions and enlightened ideas about the issue of compulsive eating and its emotional causes.

No criticism. Group members support one another. Never criticise another group member, rather try and see the good in each person. Everyone is encouraged to praise and appreciate both her own achievements and those of the other group members. Acknowledging both large and small accomplishments alike, whilst striving to overcome the addiction to food.

These guidelines help all concerned become more and more aware, conscious and successful in all areas of life.

Avoid advice giving, rather individual members share what has worked for them in similar situations.

One person talks at a time and all the other group members listen until the speaker is finished, only then sharing relevant knowledge, information or experience. (Maybe have a ten minute or fifteen minute max for each person if necessary; for sometimes there tends to be one person who 'overtakes' the group by compulsively speaking most of the time. This needs to be kept in check).

**Equal time:** The group leader, facilitator or organiser ensures that each group member has more or less equal amounts of time when speaking. Although some naturally keep quieter than others, and some will be more talkative, these too are traits to be looked at and the individual encouraged to be aware of and consider. The topics of 'being heard' and 'being listened to' are important to discuss. Did you feel 'heard' as a child? Does your husband listen to you? Questions like this are very important.

**Support:** The goal of the support group is to provide support and help each member to achieve three main objectives:
1. To eat when hungry and stop when full.
2. To pinpoint and resolve the emotional issues that trigger eating when full.

3. To raise self-acceptance.

## Food History

On your first meeting – everyone is given a pen a paper to jot down their food history. About ten or fifteen sentences on key points in their past and present experience around food, size and shape. Things such as - How long they have had the problem. If they know what their emotional triggers are. What issues can cause them to eat when full, how often they eat when full or are they totally unaware of when that fullness sensation kicks in? A key memory of a painful incident that caused them to turn to food when full.

Then one by one, everyone shares what they want to share about what they wrote. In this way we acknowledge our shared past and our commitment to ourselves and each other to create a supportive environment to heal and change.

## What would a loving supportive mother say?

A lot of us are unloved mothers – that is we are mothers ourselves yet we did not get much loving support from our own mothers when we were children. We came from a dysfunctional family. This inevitably and appropriately begs the question – How to heal the wounds from not getting enough loving support? Well the first step is open up a dialogue between the inner daughter and inner mother only this time make her a loving wise mother! Thus re-writing the original script in the places that it is abusive, unloving and unsupportive. Thus giving yourself a new healthy blueprint to work from, to live from.

When her child is frightened, what does a loving wise, supportive mother do? She listens. What does the loving wise mother say? – This is how to treat your very own self when you are afraid. Listen to your own concerns and say the wise, loving, supportive thing to yourself.

When her child says – I'm hungry – and it is half an hour before dinner, what does a loving, wise, supportive mother do and say? Say this to yourself when you are hungry half an hour before dinner.

When her child wants desert before her savoury dish, what does a loving, wise, supportive mother say? Say this to yourself when you want something sweet before savoury.

When her child is angry, what does a loving, wise, supportive mother say?

You get the idea. This exercise is not so much about getting right or wrong answers. It is asking you to look at how your inner mother talks to your inner child. It is probably a re-enactment of how your real life mother talked to you as a child. This inner dialogue can be altered and changed to a healthier one. One that lovingly supports you throughout life.

You know at times you are going to want a bowl of ice cream before lunch! And we need to look at how unimportant it is if we eat something sweet before something savoury. We need to know that it's okay to eat what we want, when we want and long as we are genuinely physically hungry and that is what we fancy eating at that moment in time. It is a natural expression of individual freedom, to allow oneself the joy of eating what you fancy when you fancy it, regardless of the time of day, or its calorie content, because you trust yourself that overall you have a healthy balanced nutritious food intake that happens to involve ice-cream before lunch sometimes. I speak from experience here!

Now a word to the critics - I am not condoning gluttony. We are working on eliminating the compulsive eating, the eating when physically full. The eating that is done, not out of genuine physical hunger, but the eating that is done to suppress emotions. The eating that is the direct cause of excess weight. Remember – Eating when physically full causes excess weight over and above the type of foods you eat.

It is in denying ourselves the foods we fancy when physically hungry that we plant the seed of a full blown binge. In order to effectively deal with this compulsion to binge, the elimination of any sense of deprivation, is essential. We accomplish this solely through the constant reassurance that we can eat whatever we want, as long as we are physically hungry and that is what we fancy eating.

So to recap - You may already realise that you are responding to yourself the way your mother responded to you as a child when any issue around food or weight comes up. What I can and can't eat etc. The good news is, you can change the script. You can change your responses to you. This can help you change you repeating patterns. Maybe when you were sad your mother's response was a bar of chocolate rather than a big hug and a conversation about what caused you to feel sad. Now, in present time you may still be doing the same thing to yourself – giving yourself a bar of chocolate when you are full, when in truth you need a friend to talk to, some quiet time or a hug.

So, think of loving supportive things you like to do. Think of loving supportive things to say to yourself when you are in need of comfort. For fear, loneliness or anger consider how to deal with each of these emotions in new ways. Food when full is not the answer for dealing with these emotions, now is your time to find out what is.

Look through You Tube, self-help books, support groups or holistic therapies to find the ones you like to help you on this new journey of feeling your feelings and healing your emotional issues as you get slim and stay slim through eating when hungry and stopping when full.

## Group work

Starting or joining a self-help support group to explore the concepts in this book can be very useful. Meeting once a week either in person or on-line for support, sharing of experiences and gleaning insights and wisdom. Allow the group dynamic be a place of discovery, support, friendship and knowledge. As you ponder the issues that surface, you can resolve them both individually and within the group. Learning to listen and also learning to be heard is fundamental in any healing process of an emotional nature. We discover our own personal way of coping with feelings and emotional dilemmas, and we open up a new way of dealing with old problems with the company of others on the same path.

Sometimes a re-enactment of the mother daughter relationship will become very clear in a group. The group facilitator or another group member consciously or unconsciously represents the projecting group member's mother. Because in the group, it is a rule that we all offer only support and understanding to each other and no criticism is permitted, it produces a very supportive atmosphere. If a supportive atmosphere is not the projecting group member's normal experience there may be an adverse reaction and a subconscious desire to provoke the mother figure into reacting the same way as the real mother reacted. By 'projecting group member' I mean a group member that is projecting an image of their own mother on to another group member. Like saying – 'You will re-enact the dysfunctional dynamic that went on in my early childhood, respond to me the way my mother did, shout, criticise or belittle, so I can battel with it once again.' This is how we all behave until we gain enough conscious awareness of our own patterns of interaction and willingly heal and change that pattern to a healthier more harmonious one.

When all the projecting group member gets is continued understanding and support, she is receiving what she never got from her mother. With her raised conscious awareness she can see her pattern and allow herself to feel the unfamiliar positive dynamic of genuine friendship and emotional support. Tears may be shed. To remember and acknowledge old unpleasant memories of the past is often painful, especially if we have been avoiding them for some time.

We are all learning exactly how the dysfunctions of the past affected us and we can be reassured that we can now look at them and resolve them forever. It can bring up angry and sad feelings too. Feeling these feelings means they can be healthily integrated rather than unhealthily suppressed.

## Processing anger visualisation

Do not do this visualisation when driving or doing other things. When we feel our anger and notice its powerful energy without lashing out at anyone or having a binge on food to suppress it, we realise that this energy called anger can carry an important message. Some injustice or wrong has been done and we need purposefulness to heal it. Anger, acknowledged and processed healthily, changes into purposefulness.

The group facilitator or a group member can read the following aloud or record the following on tape, remembering to leave ample time for thoughts, images and feelings to come into awareness where the dots indicate. You can also do this visualisation on your own.

Close your eyes and imagine what it feels like to be angry… it helps to think of something or someone who makes you angry… who was that person… what did they do to make you feel angry… focus on the angry feelings and ask them – What message do you have for me…? What wrong has been done to make me feel angry…? What is the solution to this injustice…? Do I leave a person or situation…? What is the best and healthiest course of action in this situation for me to take if any…?

Notice is the feeling of anger held anywhere in your body… Does it shift and change, into sorrow for example or fear…? If so, allow yourself to feel this new emotion, again just noticing if it is held anywhere in your body… Ask your body to show you what that emotion that is held in your body looks like, does it have a colour or texture…? And what healing colour does it need to heal…? Breathe that colour into your body and visualise that healing colour filling up that area of previously stuck anger. I would like you to imagine what it feels like to be purposeful… Getting up in the morning with a purpose to be happy and healthy saying to yourself – Today is going to be a good day or use the famous healing affirmation – Every day in every way things are getting better and better for me now.

Slowly allow yourself to come back to the room, breathe deeply a couple of times, feel the chair (or floor) under you supporting you, yawn or stretch and share your experiences with the group or in a private note book if you wish.

## Integrating fear visualisation

Do not do this visualisation when driving or doing other things. Now, allow your body to relax… I would like you to feel what it is like to be afraid… Just allow yourself to experience what fear feels like for you… Remember a time when you felt afraid... Why were you afraid...? Was someone else with you...? Experience as much fear as you can knowing you can back away from it at any time if it gets too uncomfortable... Breathe deeply a few times and remind yourself you are safe now and like a brave explorer, simply exploring this feeling called fear... How does fear feel in your body, is it held in any one location in your body, such as the throat or stomach...? Know that you are in control and can handle this emotion. Now ask yourself – What do I want to do in this situation...? Do you want to leave...? Then see yourself quietly leaving, being able to leave without any problem... No one notices you and you are able to leave without objection... You keep going until you are far away from that situation and are safe... Well done!

Now I would like you to imagine that you are really enthusiastic about something. Something wonderful is about to happen, or you are involved in something you really love... Positive ideas are flowing and support to implement those ideas comes forth as well as like-minded friends to help you... Notice your positive thoughts.... If any negative thoughts slip in, they are soon counteracted with a positive solution or way forward... See yourself accomplishing your goal... See yourself getting what you want as you are feeling this great intensity of feeling... you could be accomplishing your biggest dream... How does it feel to be enthusiastic...? Notice what you are doing as you accomplish your dream with enthusiasm... How are you relating to the people around you with this enthusiasm and positivity...? Allow yourself to be guided by that enthusiasm for what you desire in life and feel yourself emersed in enthusiasm and getting the results you want with ease and in a win / win way... Slowly let the scene fade, breathe deeply a few times, yawn and stretch if you wish and jot down or share your experience and thoughts.

## Pair work and spoken affirmations for groups

The group leader asks everyone to get into pairs. Ask each to choose to be person 'A' or person 'B'.

The whole group affirms together – I now lose my excess weight easily and permanently and in peace. I now heal my emotional issues easily and permanently and in peace. I am my perfect weight now.

Then the group leader asks the 'A's to tell their 'B' partners what it is like to be slim. You can draw from actual experiences of when you were slim or you can be imagining what it would be like to be slim. Either way she states what her experiences of being slim are, and talks as if she were already slim. 'B's role in this is to just listen. The group leader watches the clock – five minutes for this one. When the five minutes is up 'A' writes down all her positive aspects of being slim. 'B' can help with this reminding 'A' of all the positive qualities 'A' mentioned being connected with slimness. Write down as many positive slim qualities as you can recall talking about.

Now it is the 'B's turn to tell the 'A's about their experiences of being slim. Again talking in the present tense as if already slim. Now it is 'A's turn to listen. The group leader again watches the clock and when five minutes have passed the 'A's write down what positive aspects their slimness gives them. Remembering as many possible with the help of 'B'.

Both now construct some I am…. affirmations with their own positive aspects of being slim. Such as, I am attractive. I am popular. I am happy.

Each chooses one affirmation and together with their partner affirm that affirmation 15 times, noticing how they feel emotionally as they affirm these statements aloud together.

The group forms a circle again and each member has a chance to talk about how that felt and what came up for them.

The purpose is, again, to focus on developing now the quality that you believe you will have once slim. The truth is you can develop any quality, have any quality now, from within yourself, no matter what your present size or shape. Affirmations are the most effective way of developing qualities and desired states such as calmness, attractiveness, more confidence or whatever it is you feel being slim has to offer.

## Twelve states of mind conducive to healing your eating habit

1. Willingness to feel your feelings.
2. Intention to feel your feelings and find new ways to deal with feelings that used to cause you to eat when full.
3. Focus on your feelings especially when you are physically full.
4. Focus on what you desire from life, relationships, health and career.

5. Persistence in using the healthy alternative tools for resolving emotional issues.
6. Belief that you can succeed. Believe in your ability to be free from compulsive eating forever. Author's note: Sometimes I look at my life and what I am working on accomplishing seems to be three steps ahead of me in terms of my ability, or in terms of possibility. Only to find that it is possible and I have the capability as I believe and persist. I discover the strength, talent, ability and resourcefulness, reveal themselves to me as I exercise my faith in my abilities by doing whatever it is that I decided to accomplish.
7. Awareness of your feelings and emotional issues.
8. Gentleness towards yourself and others.
9. Kindness towards yourself and others.
10. Acceptance of yourself and others.
11. Forgiveness of yourself and others. See: howardwills.com
12. Responsibility for yourself and your actions and experiences of past and present.

In abiding by these aforementioned states of mind you will nurture yourself and in so doing you will be all the more able to nurture your loved ones and accept nurturing from others too.

**Vitamins and minerals**
You may wonder how you are supposed to ensure a healthy, well-balanced food intake, with all this focusing on emotional issues and self-acceptance going on. The answer lies in the subtle

cues our bodies are giving us all the time, regardless of whether we listen to them or not. One of the major guidelines for natural, permanent weight loss is, eat when you are genuinely physically hungry and stop when you are genuinely physically full. Within this guideline is the concept – Listen to your body. As you tune inwards, listen to and respond appropriately to when your stomach is physically hungry or full. You also become aware of the fine-tuning which tells you degrees of hunger and fullness. The various sensations which include starving-hungry, positively stuffed and all the in-betweens become clearer and clearer to you, until you know, without a shadow of a doubt, exactly when to eat, how much to eat and when to stop eating. It becomes automatic. Also when genuinely physically hungry you get to know whether you fancy something savoury or sweet, orange juice or water, vegetables or fruit, meat or vegan products etc. It is amazing to know that when your body fancies orange juice it is it's way of telling you it needs vitamin C! If you want meat or red kidney bean stew, it is telling you that that is what it needs to satisfy its nutritional needs. Trusting the simplicity of the body ensures all your nutritional needs are met. Of course you can consult the experts or seek out information online about what foods contain what minerals and vitamins, take supplements, superfoods and look into detoxing. This is all helpful and if you are basically being drawn to healthy foods and are keeping sugars, alcohol, and carbs to a minimum; and feel like you have enough energy then you are on the right track. As always follow your intuition over and above anything else. Your gut instinct will tell you what is right for you at any individual moment in time.

## Think slim

Once you have established the healthy habit of eating what you want when physically hungry, always stopping when physically full, resolving your emotional issues and maintaining a high level of self-acceptance, you are well on the way to a complete recovery. After all, these are the three major keys which, operating together, actually allow the body to find and maintain its own natural weight. Natural, permanent weight loss is inevitable at this stage. One of the final steps which you can take now, to help you mentally accept your slimmer-self is to think slim. Thinking slim can be done at any stage of recovery from overeating, but is particularly useful at this end stage where you are starting to actually lose the excess weight.

What are you thinking when slim? Example: You are standing at the bus stop on your way to work, or in line at the supermarket and while you wait, you think to yourself – I have already lost all the excess weight and I am now as slim as I dreamed of being. Notice how it feels. Is it scary? Do you feel in any way vulnerable or uncomfortable? Is it very joyous and you feel a bit ungrounded and too light so to speak. Just feel the feelings, notice them, think of how you can address them, what can you do to ground yourself or help you experience this intensity of new feeling? Allow the feelings to be felt and allow them to pass.

Thinking slim can be done as soon as you wake up. Think to yourself – I have done it! I am now my slim self and I have lost all the weight! Again notice how it feels as you imagine yourself slim in this present moment. Do you feel good about yourself? Are you still bogged down with the same problems you had yesterday? If so, acceptance is the key, knowing that the slim you may still have problems and issues, but you now have the power to not overeat because of those issues. You go on with your day. What do you wear or consider wearing as you pretend to be slim, as you think slim, is it new clothes and different style? Notice how they feel these new clothes and different styles. Maybe they are not so comfortable and not something you want to wear fat or slim. This is a discovery you can make at the larger size before you get slim and can thus not be ambushed by these uncomfortable feelings at the smaller size. Realise and resolve them now at the larger size as you think slim.

Most of you will already be feeling the wonderful sense of relief and inner well-being as a direct result of having replaced an old addicted relationship to food with a new healthier non-addicted one, and are enjoying the fullness of what that means. Experiencing that new precious quality that your life now contains, embraces the return of what you thought you had lost but had only forgotten for a short time – a strong awareness of and respect for your body, your feelings and your hunger and fullness sensations. You have done well and journeyed far. Returning home from your painful and dissatisfying wanderings into suppression and addiction. Home at last to familiar and clear ways of truth and love. The most important truth, the most important love. The truth about body size, eating habits and love for yourself. Thank goodness! I appreciate you for your commitment to your own healing. Thank you for taking the journey of personal growth which you and many others have taken, for in so doing you are making your life and the planet even more wonderful!

## Thoughts on a hot afternoon

The day is hot, about noon and all is well. My continued spiritual study, and in particular my practice of 'The Course in Miracles' offers me more and more each day. I can literally feel the increased amounts of joy, understanding, patience, love, forgiveness and security that are welling up from within me. The positive spin-offs of this increase are harmony and love such as never before. Peace, established in every area of my life and a feeling that I am doing something positive to help myself and others to a more loving, natural, happy and secure life. The lessons I have learned in the last ten years have been priceless and precious. I gained tools from reading books and meeting people. These tools when applied to any situation that bothers me, enables me to see that situation in a positive light. A light, which allows, everyone concerned to grow and be positively enlightened even healed. I myself have experienced much healing in those ten years and much positive change and growth. I have had backsliding and sometimes hard, sad and frightening times, out of which emerged a desire stronger than I, which pushed me to search for the answer, to search for the reason, to search for the good. The doorway out of those difficult times always appeared and led me to more and more doorways to self-development and growth. All of these doors, I discovered the key to and opened sometimes joyously, sometimes nervously, sometimes with fear and sometimes with just sheer determination to see what was on the other side. Always enlightened, strengthened, encouraged and inspired by both the process and the results. I wish enlightenment for every human being on this beautiful earth of ours. Have the life you want to have. Be the person you want to be. Plan, persist and believe in yourself. Grow, heal prosper and be blessed for the answers and ability are all within you. Develop and allow yourself to see your inner dreams reflected in your outer world.

## Conclusion

So what now? You have healed your eating disorder. You are eating when you are hungry and stopping when you are full. You resolve your emotional issues rather than suppressing them. You feel your feelings allowing them to be your guides. You can say to yourself – I accept my size and shape exactly as it is right now. I pinpoint and resolve my emotional stuff no matter what. And believe it! When you reach this stage, I say continue. If there were one word I would encourage you to take with you, it would be – vigilance. Fundamentally, vigilance is of the utmost importance now.

## Be vigilant

Be vigilant for the cravings and compulsions, dismiss them and stay centred. Be true to yourself, your feelings and values, for thus you can learn, heal and be guided to peace. Allow your values evolve. Have faith in your values, in what you believe to be true. Believe your gut instincts, for they speak the truth. Obey and follow your feelings of joy. Heed your feelings of anxiety, fear and anger for they too have a message of guidance to offer. Do not be afraid to ask what that message is, or to act on it. For this message gives you added insights into the nature of every situation in which you may find yourself, and inspirational hints about how to deal with each one.

As you connect with your true self, you learn much and are protected as you stay aware. Thus you have your alternative to addiction and obsession. This is a new way of dealing with whatever life has in store for you. And so you are empowered to create the life you truly wish for and deserve. You start to chase your dreams, making them your priority, your focus of attention and intention. Satisfaction and fulfilment come your way and stay, even in among the challenges that may appear, to be dealt with.

Be vigilant for times when you know you are distancing yourself from your feelings and the potential for addictive tendencies to take over your habits and your life. The enemy within, that's addiction. Watch out for it. It can appear anywhere in your life and usually where you least expect. It can wear a disguise and trick you. If you have an unresolved feeling or emotional issue and you avoid it, beware, for you may find it crops up in your finances, health or relationships. You may even find yourself getting angry or anxious to avoid your pain or fear. Do not be ashamed. Be vigilant and know that it is not only okay to ask for help with unresolved emotional stuff, but it is essential! For to dive into the unpleasant waters of the subconscious in order to fish out and resolve its suppressed contents, takes skill and bravery. It is good to have a helping hand whilst accomplishing such a task. You only have to fish in these subconscious depths a few times and resolve a few issues to be convinced that later rewards are no less than fabulous. The once murky sea of subconscious negativity becomes crystal clear, from healing love, and inner peace. May this be your truth.

A final word: Vigilance implies the sacred as when one holds a vigil. Also it has connotations of war or warlike conditions. People in war situations, soldiers and warriors have to be vigilant for the enemy. The enemy here is cravings. Real warriors bring something sacred to the battle. The recovering and recovered compulsive eater alike, needs to know the sacredness of her life now she is bidding to be free (or actually free from) addiction to food when full. She needs to know she is something of a vigilante, a peaceful warrior, aware of the truth, aware that the danger from addiction is real and that dissolving her own inner enemy, her cravings, is her responsibility on her path to establishing and maintaining ultimate well-being.

For further information on Sofia's workshops, books and one to one sessions:
Email: sofia2227@gmail.com
Phone / Text: 07530 531 655
Facebook: Sofia Bothwell
Instagram: author_sofia22
Web: www.sofiabothwell.co.uk
Blog: sofiabothwell.blogspot.com

Sofia Bothwell

Printed and bound by CPI Group (UK) Ltd, Croydon, CR0 4YY

12/06/2025

01900232-0001